WHAT OTHERS ARE SAYING ABOUT
BROKEN BREAD

"It's easy to spot our cultural obsession with food. We have TV shows featuring cooking competitions, documentaries explaining the hidden dangers in our food, and bookstores packed with every type of cookbook situated alongside the latest and greatest lifestyle diet books. In her new book, *Broken Bread: How to Stop Using Food and Fear to Fill Spiritual Hunger*, Tilly Dillehay considers how our various sin struggles with food—from gluttony to snobbery—can overflow in guilt, judgement, anxiety, or pride as we contemplate a simple question: What's for dinner? She writes with conviction and compassion as she directs our eyes to a better and more-needed spiritual feast—one truly able to satisfy and sustain our daily lives."

Melissa Kruger,
TGC Director of Women's Initiatives and author of *Growing Together*

"This is a book Christian women need—at least the ones who eat food. Tilly helps us see that food idolatry comes in more than one form. She carefully helps us diagnose our sin problem regarding food, and she then points us to food's rightful place and purpose in our lives. Read this book if you want to have peace with God and peace with what you eat."

Abigail Dodds,
author of *(A)Typical Woman* and contributor at Desiring God

"*Broken Bread* is an intelligent and biblical discussion of food issues. It's a massive table covered with dishes of wisdom right out of the oven, which are enhanced with the brown gravy of good sense and set out before an emaciated people who have been suffering through a famine."

Douglas Wilson,
...rch, Moscow, Idaho

BROKEN BREAD

TILLY DILLEHAY

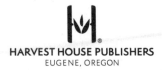

HARVEST HOUSE PUBLISHERS
EUGENE, OREGON

Cover design by Studio Gearbox

Cover photo © jamesteohart, Nor Gal / Shutterstock; Yaroslav Danylchenko / Stocksy

Interior design by Angie Renich / Wildwood Digital Publishing

Broken Bread
Copyright © 2020 by Tilly Dillehay
Published by Harvest House Publishers
Eugene, Oregon 97408
www.harvesthousepublishers.com

ISBN 978-0-7369-8013-5 (pbk)
ISBN 978-0-7369-8014-2 (eBook)

Library of Congress Cataloging-in-Publication Data is on file at the Library of Congress, Washington, DC.

Printed in the United States of America

20 21 22 23 24 25 26 27 28/ BP-AR / 10 9 8 7 6 5 4 3 21

CONTENTS

For Justin first of all,
and Norah, Agnes, and Henry next of all.

It's a privilege to cook for you and eat with you.

The Four Food Poles

The woman in front of me turned back to hand me a Styrofoam plate she'd just pried loose from the stack. It was a small gesture of hospitality, one that would become familiar to me over the years to come. I took it and awkwardly moved down the row, feeling that all eyes were on me as I plopped a wedge of meatloaf, a piece of home-made bread, and a small pile of salad on my plate.

All eyes were most emphatically not on me, but as the Proverb goes, the wicked flee when no one pursues. I had lived in the shad-ows for so long, I couldn't even navigate a church potluck without flinching. As I slid into a white plastic chair in front of a white plas-tic table next to the one girl I knew, I felt myself stiffening, prepar-ing for the difficulty of friendly conversation.

They all knew what I was, I felt certain of that. They knew I was a refugee from the city, a "problem case" for the pastor/biblical coun-selor. They knew that I was recalcitrant, raised in a Christian fam-ily, a self-described agnostic. But they didn't necessarily know how hungry I was—hungry in my very bones—to see what an ordi-nary Christian community might look like in a small town where the coolness factor was low. After a few years of being spiritually on the run, moving among unbelievers who served themselves openly while looking for salvation among the leaves of marijuana and between the sheets of friends, I was ready to be reminded of how ordinary Christians lived.

The people at the church potluck didn't know whose bed I had just tumbled out of a few days earlier; they didn't know that I was caught in a cycle of overeating and throwing up food. They didn't know that the shame of food and the shame of sexuality felt somehow intertwined for me—both were things to enjoy in secret, with consequences that humbled you in public. They only knew that I had a lost look on my face, that it was lunchtime and I needed a plate, that I was from out of town and needed a friendly conversation.

They also didn't know about the condescension I carried into the potluck. I assumed that these people, with their meat-and-three sensibilities, would be impressed by the refinement I brought from Nashville. It was satisfying to my limping ego to feel that, at least here, I wasn't a small fish in a big pond. I wrote about it in my journal that night, funny stories about the 72-year-old man in the blue polyester suit, comments about the quaint hymns being sung, observations about the young people in the church who seemed so unaware of the wild doings of the world outside.

But I was converted that week, sitting under that biblical counseling and hearing the gospel with ears that God had prepared for 22 years. Twenty-two years. For 22 years of sitting under good expositional preaching with parents who loved me and taught me. The ground had been prepared and seeds dropped in constantly, and yet it was in this tiny town with a church potluck every single Sunday, living as a guest in the home of ordinary believers, that God chose to whisper life into the seed and call it up from the ground.

Food continued to linger in the background of the rocky early years after my conversion. The bulimia kept stealing my time and attention. Food and cooking seemed emblematic of my ineptitude in every area of life. My condescension melted as I realized that in the small country church were cultured people—well-read, well-traveled, capable of bringing much more than a meat-and-three to the church potluck. Among them, I felt like a clumsy child trying to pretend I was a Christian adult. Hospitality was the great blessing that allowed me to move to the small town permanently—living first with one family, then with another while I got my sea legs. I grew, got a job I loved, married, started having children, and as life stages gave way to other life stages, I learned to cook. I began practicing hospitality.

My husband became a pastor in the same church, and food still lingered in my life, only this time it was behind the ministry work we were doing. It began to represent something besides shame and social clout to me. I began to experience food as something else: a good gift from God and a tool in my hand. It became a means of grace.

But the complications of food still intruded themselves on my own life at times. I still spent time in the ditches of gluttony, snobbery, apathy, and asceticism. And friends of mine often talked about the ways food complicated their lives. I watched friends become allergic to gluten, only to become unallergic a few years later. One young mother posted online about the struggles of dieting without becoming obsessed, and I was amazed by the well-meaning comments from other Christians: "Think of food as just fuel for life," "You are what you eat!" and "I just think of food in two categories— poison and medicine." A lady at church told me of her hurt feelings when her daughter-in-law came for dinner the first and only time and was unable to eat the meal served because she was doing keto.

I started to root around for books that celebrated eating as a gift from God and explored these sticky topics of taking care of our bodies without being driven around by the winds of diet culture. I found precious little. The flavors I'd experienced at the church potluck—the gospel flavors of hospitable love, simplicity, and patient fellowship with people from many different culinary backgrounds—were not easy to find in the Christian bookstore. Some of the most straightforward commands in Scripture about food were often unexamined in the literature, passed over in favor of repeated examinations of 1 Corinthians 6:19 ("Or do you not know that your body is a temple of the Holy Spirit within you, whom you have from God?").

It felt to me like the zeitgeist of twenty-first century American culture, with its unique food anxieties, was controlling the way we spoke, wrote, and practiced. Most importantly, it felt to me like we were being untrue to the larger picture presented in the Word of God, distracted by a moment in time.

The Complicating Factors

Food is complicated for so many good reasons. It's complicated by our sin and by our bodily afflictions in a fallen world. It is complicated by scarcity, and it is complicated by plenty. It is complicated by social pressure and pride. It's complicated by gluttony and by asceticism. It's complicated by advertising. It's complicated by economic forces. It's complicated by the fact that even though Jesus and Paul tell us that we aren't contaminated by what goes into the body but by what comes out of it, our default approach to physical things is to assume that the stricter the rule, the holier the person.

We Christian women are idolatrous and confused and fearful, even while we are skilled, hospitable, and self-sacrificing. In the church, our food issues look entirely too much like the food issues of the world around us. In this, as in every other personal practice, we have a great opportunity to model freedom and generosity. We have a great opportunity to bring the joy of Christ into our kitchens, as we are bringing him into our bedrooms, bathrooms, living rooms, libraries, front yards, backyards, and neighborhoods.

"When I talk with older saints that weathered the storms of yesteryear," writes Doug Ponder, "they speak in unison about this cultural moment: The frequency and intensity of the focus on food today far surpasses the culinary concerns of the past. It would seem that social media, plus the internet, plus blog culture, plus fitness magazines, plus hypersexual entertainment, plus restaurant trends, plus alternative health movements minus a robustly biblical view of food is a powerful cocktail that's polluting the hearts of millions."[1]

God cares about how we eat. He cares much more about how we eat than he cares about what we eat.[2]

Let that sink in for a moment. If you have been treating food like a burden to be carried for the family or a rule book to be followed or a club with which to beat yourself, this sounds counterintuitive. *God doesn't care what you eat? But how will I care for my temple?*

Be patient with me, and you'll see what I mean when I say God doesn't care what you eat. He has (almost) said as much, as we'll see.

Four Food Poles

If I was going to attach diagnoses to the main food sins I see in the church, they'd come down to four: asceticism, gluttony, snobbery, and apathy. I've been mixed up in each of these, one at a time or several at a time. Think of them as two sets of twin vices: asceticism versus gluttony, and snobbery versus apathy.

Asceticism is being "too proud to enjoy the enjoyable" according to J.I. Packer. It is a belief that God is as stingy as we are, and a fundamental distrust of anything that is too enjoyable, too luxurious, too free, too unstructured. We find strict diets attractive because we are, in our hearts, very ready to believe that anything fun is probably bad. This is where you find Christians who want to bring back dietary laws stricter than the ones Jesus did away with at his coming. Asceticism loves rules and distrusts freedom. It views food as either a medicine to be swallowed ("food will heal you") or a tool to be used in survival ("food is just fuel").

Gluttony is on the opposite pole from asceticism. Gluttony is simple, straightforward, and easy to diagnose. It cannot be satisfied. It's unsatisfied at the end of a delicious, sit-down meal. It's unsatisfied in front of the TV. It's unsatisfied at the all-you-can-eat buffet. It wants to taste everything in rapid succession. It busts out of any limitation placed on it—always wanting more. We want salty because we just ate sweet; we want sweet because we just ate salty. Gluttony is one of those sins of the flesh that gains strength the more it is fed. It's antithetical to self-control. It is also a great foundation upon which to build the ascetic's fear of food.

Snobbery wants to make our friends feel behind because they've never heard of yacon syrup. (I've never heard of this myself until I just now googled "food fads 2019," so I can only assume it's something really egregious, like a cross between bacon and yams.) Snobbery is consumed with being on the right side of food history. This is a social sin—one that is acted out mostly in front of others on social media or over the supper table. Love trumps dietary restrictions, according to Paul's letter to the Corinthians. But food snobbery, when given free rein, trumps love.

On the opposite pole from snobbery, you find apathy. **Apathy** digs in its heels and refuses to believe that any objective fault could be found with the McDonald's McRib sandwich. Food apathy can't be bothered to learn to cook. It is too lazy to think about it. Apathy leads us to miss out on the breathtaking array of sights, smells, and tastes that God has laid out on the global table. We live in an era that offers astounding culinary variety, and offers it to the average middle-class person with access to a kitchen and a grocery store. Apathy sniffs at this and continues to subsist on Hungry Man frozen dinners.

Idolatry in Its Many Forms

These food poles are all just different iterations of a food idol. They are each an attempt to use physical food to fill a spiritual hunger—hunger for righteousness, for pleasure, for significance, or for ease.

I have taken my turn at each of these modes of food worship. I have used rules to try to stop the runaway horse of gluttony. I have used food fads to try to stave off feelings of insignificance among my fellow humans. I have pulled away and tried to just not think about any of it because decisions are too hard and knowledge brings responsibility.

In the end, I still bump around from pole to pole for seasons at a time. But as I grow in the Lord, as I continue to feed people besides myself, and as I begin to divorce my measurement of righteousness from what I ate for lunch, I continue to experience new freedom, growth, and joy.

If bread could be used to tempt Jesus, then I imagine that it can be used to tempt me. No servant is greater than his master (John 13:16). He is teaching me slowly that I don't live by bread alone, but by every word that comes from the mouth of God (Matthew 4:4). He's teaching me that what goes into my mouth can't contaminate me—that distinction is reserved for what comes out of my mouth (Matthew 15:11).

So what can we do? We love the food, we hate the food, we want to eat the food, and we want to reject it. We are obsessed and fearful, prideful and lazy. How shall we Christians learn to eat? How shall we learn that whether we eat or drink we can do it to the glory of God (1 Corinthians 10:31)?

In this book, I want to wade into all of these questions. They're full of important nuances, they're relevant to our lives, and I believe they're something that our Savior cares about deeply.

PART 1

FOUR POLES

CHAPTER 1

Food Is Fuel

ASCETICISM AT THE TABLE

> We must therefore reject different varieties, which engender various mischiefs...that of cookery, and the useless art of making pastry. For people dare to call by the name of food their dabbling in luxuries, which glides into mischievous pleasures.[1]
>
> —CLEMENT OF ALEXANDRIA

From Memory: 2002

I am 14. I am standing in the family kitchen in Hermitage, Tennessee, fishing frozen shrimp out of a bag and floating them in a bowl of water. The burner is on, and I'm putting a little butter in a non-stick pan.

My back is sticky from the 6:00 a.m. local YMCA spin class. I'm wearing a slick, sky-blue sleeveless shirt that I bought at Walmart with matching biker shorts that have a blue stripe on the side. I bought these things because the adult attendees of the serious 6:00 a.m. spin class wear things that look similar. My sister Sophie is 16, and she drives us, although I often have to push her out of bed.

I feel a familiar salty, crusty film over my forehead, and it is as satisfying as the quick, oxygenated feeling in my legs, the beginnings of muscular stiffness. I want to go and take over something somewhere.

I feel that I could ace a test right now or have a conversation with a total stranger without flinching. I feel invincible.

Each shrimp is dirty gray, and once I squeeze the tail and pry the shell off, I can see through its translucent skin. There's a dark thread of what I've been told is shrimp intestine running down the middle. Sometimes I pull these out because they're gross. Sometimes I leave them because I'm in a rush. There are 12 shrimp in the bowl—I counted them. Shrimp are a fatless protein luxury, and I know I'm lucky to be allowed to eat them.

I drop them, still wet from the defrosting water, into the pan. The color change is fascinating—it's the way I imagine the change when Narnia's enchanted stone creatures are turned back to life. Dark-gray shrimp slowly and perceptibly get pink as the heat is applied to them—so one side can be pink with the other side gray. Or, you can watch through a glass cover as they steam evenly and achieve a total transformation in just a few seconds.

Shrimp can get a wonderful browned exterior if you do them right. I turn them and warm up half a cup of precooked brown rice, because that is what the man from *Body for Life* said to do. One palm size of protein, one palm size of acceptable carbs. I am 14, and I am on fire for this diet.

I sit at the table with a glass plate and enjoy each bite of the shrimp first. Each shrimp is like a little curl of pure seafood flavor, with a lingering sensation of salt butter. Biting through each one is like biting through a very thick balloon, if the balloon were to give way instantly to your teeth. It delivers a rubbery sensation, but at the same time, a melting one.

Shrimp is wonderful.

The brown rice is plain except for a little salt and pepper. I don't enjoy it. But I eat it because that is what the *Body for Life* man said to do. And I'm not going to lose those five pounds by disobeying the *Body for Life* man.

"Eat, and live," says the *Body for Life* man.

Holy Corn Flakes

It was May of 1866. Ellen White stood and gave a presentation to a relatively new group: the Seventh-Day Adventists. She said she'd received a word from God, and it was a word about food.

God had drawn her attention to Genesis, the verse where he gives Adam and Eve "every herb bearing seed, which is upon the face of all the earth, and every tree, in the which is the fruit of a tree yielding seed; to you it shall be for meat" (Genesis 1:29, KJV).

She announced to the group that this verse was a command—a command to live off of plants exclusively. She told her flock that not only should they abstain from meat but also from tobacco, coffee, tea, and alcohol. She warned against excessive spicy condiments, against salt and pickled foods, against overeating and frying, against using any kind of drug, and against wearing then-ubiquitous corsets and tight dresses. She warned that sensual indulgences like spicy food, meat, and tobacco led to the sins of masturbation and excessive sexual intercourse.

Not long after Ellen White's edict, she and her husband took a young man named John Harvey Kellogg under their wing. They hired him to run the printer and eventually to edit the Seventh-Day Adventist's primary evangelistic vehicle, which was a health advice magazine called *The Health Reformer*. The young man soon found that he had a talent for writing and marketing.

They sent him to medical school. He came back to Battle Creek in 1876 and formed the Battle Creek Sanitarium, which was soon known all over the world. It was a grand hotel, spa, and medical center. John and his younger brother Will ran this business, and at its peak it saw between 12,000 and 15,000 patients a year.

Dr. Kellogg saw that the American people suffered with indigestion and spent too much time cooking basic food like breakfast grains. He decided he needed to create a healthy, attractive food that was easy to prepare and easy on the digestive system. He and his brother experimented with baking grains at very high heats to break down their starches—what he called "dextrinization." This was how they invented breakfast cereal. It's how we got Kellogg's Corn Flakes.

Kellogg's nutritional theory may have been flawed, but the flaw in his theological system was far graver. Like Ellen White, he believed food laws could lead to righteousness. He believed what enters the body can make a man unclean—despite the fact that the Lord Jesus specifically addressed this idea: "Do you not see that whatever goes into a person from outside cannot defile him, since it enters not his heart but his stomach, and is expelled?" (Mark 7:18-19).

Contrast that statement from Jesus with Kellogg's interpretation of a passage from Matthew 11:

> Said the great Teacher, "If your son asks for bread, will you give him a stone?" The body calls for bread, for life-giving food, but how often we supply, instead, such indigestible, unwholesome rubbish as pickles, green olives, fried foods, and various abominable mixtures which bring into the body death rather than life. How often, too, the voice which calls for pure, life-giving water is insanely answered by such disease-producing drinks as beer, whisky, wine, tea, or coffee, and the like.[2]

Kellogg, reading these precious words from Jesus about how God feeds and cares for us, could only see a lesson on the dangers of pickles and green olives. Jesus ushered in a new era for Israelite

ceremonial law, fulfilling and updating it to reflect the inaugura-
tion of his kingdom. Among his many clarifying, life-giving statements, Jesus made this statement about food and sin: *Nothing can
defile you by going into your mouth. Sin, from inside the heart, is what
defiles you.*

Kellogg, on the other hand, faced with the health struggles of
his time, decided that some foods could, indeed, defile you. There
were holy foods and unholy foods. Life-giving foods and foods that
bring death. He fashioned new food laws for his followers, following the directives of his teacher, Ellen White, rather than the "great
Teacher," Jesus Christ.

Paul encouraged the Corinthians, "Food will not commend us
to God. We are no worse off if we do not eat, and no better off if we
do" (1 Corinthians 8:8). But Kellogg made a living off of the idea
that food could, in fact, commend you to God.

He understood something about human nature. Where you find
people, you find religious people. You find people who are hard-
wired for worship, people who are afraid of dying and who long to
regain a sense of control over life. And some of these people can be
sold a religious dietary package. They will buy a religion that promises life in return for culinary devotion (complete with a righteous
rejection of green olives—or sugar, or wheat, or meat, or dairy, or
carbs, or fat, or alcohol, or caffeine, or happiness).[3]

Taking Turns as Kellogg

All of us have been Kellogg at one time or another. I know almost
no human woman in my acquaintance who hasn't taken a turn at
this.

At some point in our lives, we have assembled for ourselves a
white list and a black list of foods. We assemble them from books.
We assemble them from things we picked up among our friends.

We assemble them from the labels in the grocery aisles. We assemble them (heaven help us) from the internet.

On the white list are foods that have promised to make us attractive and young. They are superfoods. They are clean foods. Depending on our sources, they may be foods with labels that proclaim "fat free," "sugar free," "gluten free," "dairy free," "cholesterol free," or "organic." They are safe foods. They're expensive foods, much of the time.

The black list contains sugar and processed carbs. The black list contains animal products and oil. The black list contains bread and salt and nightshades and foods that feed candida microbes. Alcohol. Grains of any kind. Anything raw. Anything cooked. Anything grown by industrial farms. Anything that looks icky. Anything that tastes good. Anything besides apples and white rice (a girl I read about years ago subsisted on nothing but these two foods for several years). Anything with cloven hooves that doesn't chew the cud (Leviticus 11:1-3).

Many of us have also experienced seasonal shifts in our list. Our black list may contain one thing for six months, only to be replaced by something quite different and even contradictory for the six months following. The changes are exhausting to us and to our families, but we can't-stop-won't-stop. We're not well yet. Not thin yet. Not happy yet. The promises we've been given—about new, transformed selves and lives—have not yet been fulfilled.

In the process, Christ-followers though we are, we overlook our bondage to the teachings of the world. We are entirely too dependent on the ideas of worldly minds—minds that are still on the hunt for a Bread of Life (John 6:35). Or, if we prefer the Christian bookstore version of these doctrines, we become dependent on the teachings of Christians who write new food laws for us.

We are Christian women, but it is hard to distinguish our

experiences with food from the experiences of our unbelieving friends and family members. They, too, keep white lists and black lists. They, too, are motivated by fear of fat and fear of death. They, too, show up at dinner and say, "Oh, I'm not doing [fill in the blank] right now."

Christ broke his body for us, and ever since then, Christians ought to have been breaking bread with thanksgiving in remembrance of him. But in an age when our food problems are the problems of plenty, we have capitulated to the spirit of the age. Fear—not joy—marks our tables.

We are not guarding our hearts closely enough against this fear, which our Lord already came to eradicate. We say that we're being diligent, and we vaguely allude to passages about keeping our temples pure. But we are not applying passages that may be much more relevant to what's going on in our hearts:

- "For you did not receive the spirit of slavery to fall back into fear, but you have received the Spirit of adoption as sons, by whom we cry, 'Abba! Father!'" (Romans 8:15).

- "For God gave us a spirit not of fear but of power and love and self-control" (2 Timothy 1:7).

- "Since therefore the children share in flesh and blood, he himself likewise partook of the same things, that through death he might destroy the one who has the power of death, that is, the devil, and deliver all those who through fear of death were subject to lifelong slavery" (Hebrews 2:14-15).

Jesus delivers us not only from death but from the fear of death. Why would we want to go back? We have received the Spirit of adoption! Of power and love and self-control! Are we now to go back to fearing death—like slaves? Like people who don't have a death-defying Savior?

Our Laws and Their Laws

Peter, one of the Twelve, had a crazy vision one day at lunchtime—all the animals he'd never been allowed to eat floating toward him in a white hammock. A Voice told him to rise and kill and eat, and he protested, and then the Voice told him not to call unclean what God had declared clean.

A little while later, Peter had to swallow a much bigger piece of information. Gentiles, it turned out, were going to be part of God's family. Diet and bloodline had always been monitored rather closely under the Mosaic law, so it was a tough moment for Peter when he had to deal with the wild truth that now people of every color were going to share the broken body of Christ together.

In Peter's vision, Jesus declared freedom from a different set of laws than those most of us are operating under. For early Jewish Christians, food was still mixed up in God's good law for his people. And for early Gentile Christians, food was also mixed up in pagan idolatry. You can see why the early church felt that the question of food was a grave one.

The food laws we deal with are perhaps less grave. They usually have to do with bodily health rather than explicit command. They are more informed by the science we love so much and the opinions of influential people than by God's law. But when we read words from Jesus, Paul, and Peter—about how food can't commend us to God, can't defile us, and should no longer be weighed down with moral significance (1 Corinthians 8:8; Mark 7:19; Romans 14:14)—is there any reason why we can't apply them too?

After all, which of these systems is more substantial? The Israelite sacrificial system, or the constantly rotating system of diet restrictions you live under? If early Christians could let go of weighty religious reasons for avoiding food—to embrace Christian freedom and thanksgiving—why can't we let go of our own (arguably, less important) reasons for restricting it? Here's the bottom line: If they were free, why can't we be? If the apostles recognized that food was now a secondary matter, a matter for the conscience to navigate in the power of the Holy Spirit, why can't we?

Early Christians took the business of breaking of bread together seriously. They broke bread as a sacrament, as Jesus had directed. They broke bread as fellowship, growing the faith and growing the bonds of love. They ate freely of what had previously been forbidden, but gave preference to those with captive consciences. They guarded their hearts against gluttony, using the oil of gladness to wash down humble repast. They avoided both drunkenness (Ephesians 5:18) and the doctrines of demons ("Do not taste, Do not handle, Do not touch") (Colossians 2:21; see also 1 Timothy 4:1-5). They used the table to build community and spread the gospel.

For the first time, God's people had no food laws to prevent their sharing tables with those of other nationalities. In fact, God's people were now a quilted network of bloodlines. Food was no longer a means of division—no longer a curtain. The temple curtain had become a tablecloth, and the table was laid with Christ the Son.

Religious Eating in Postreligious Culture

Apparently, our hearts miss the food laws. They must, because we keep trying to bring them back.

Fly over 2,000 years of church history, and you arrive in twenty-first-century Western culture. Here, for the first time ever, the question is no longer "Will I eat today?" but "*What* will I eat today? Where will I buy it? How much will I eat of it?" This unusual problem is what Michael Pollan calls "the omnivore's dilemma."[4] For the first time in history, the ordinary majority doesn't scratch their living out of backyard crops of grains and root vegetables. They aren't dealing with the diseases of malnutrition. Finally, they are dealing with the diseases of plenty.

Religion and food are still linked. But now the keepers of the religious rites are members of secular religious sects. *Science can keep us alive,* declare the leaders of one sect. *Food is medicine, and it can keep us alive,* declare leaders of another sect.

The strange thing about people who bear the name of Christ is that we seem just as susceptible to this line of thinking as the non-Christian. In fact, some of us may be among the loudest voices in this chorus, except that our words are slightly different: *God can keep us alive...if we eat the right food.*

We ask questions that are so close to being good questions they're perhaps even more dangerous. Sylvester Graham, Kellogg's predecessor and inventor of the graham cracker, had this plausible-sounding objection to eating meat: "How can a man serve God with a stomach full of grease?"[5] (How indeed?)

Like the Grahams and Kelloggs of the world, we use the language of nutritional atonement, nutritional redemption, nutritional life everlasting. It's language that we don't seem to realize is directly borrowed from the world. It's also directly contradictory to the glorious fact of blood-purchased atonement, redemption, and life everlasting.

Claims from Christians writing diet books range from the believable to bizarre. "Because Jesus and people around Him ate a mostly plant-based diet with little red meat, there's little mention of 'constipation' in the bible," write A.J. Jacobs and Dr. Don Colbert.[6] Later, they add, "The key to eating like Jesus is making lunch your biggest meal and eat in as much of a relaxed atmosphere as possible."

Reese Dubin writes in *Miracle Cures from the Bible*:

What is the Bible telling us when it mentions certain foods again and again? I believe the message is clear: These are Bible Healing foods—use them, and many of your problems will vanish...cataracts, gallstones, bleeding gums, pleurisy, epilepsy, sciatica, stomach and intestinal problems, skin problems, vaginal infection, arthritis, infertility, herpes, even medicines that—thousands of years later—fight AIDS![7]

Jordan Rubin writes in *The Maker's Diet*:

> While I make no claims to offer you a "cure-all", I believe this book was inspired by God and that the practical protocol it contains can greatly improve your health. The Maker has given me a program for vibrant health based on His Word...the health principles on which this program is based are essentially the same—yesterday, today and forever. (See Hebrews 13:8.) You too can enjoy the robust health and freedom from disease by simply following the health plan designed by our Creator.[8]

Freedom from disease? Sounds like a cure-all to me. Also, it is interesting that Rubin quotes this verse from Hebrews 13:8 ("Jesus Christ is the same yesterday and today and forever") but makes no comment on the verse immediately following: "Do not be led away by diverse and strange teachings, for it is good for the heart to be strengthened by grace, not by foods, which have not benefited those devoted to them" (Hebrews 13:9).

Rubin and others like him suggest a kind of salvation via abstinence. He claims that avoiding sugar, white flour, and vegetable oils is the will of God. "Today I am on a mission from God to change people's lives and give them the message of hope and healing. I will spend the rest of my life telling the world the truth that will set them free,"[9] Rubin writes. Later, it becomes clear what the "truth that will

set them free" actually is, according to Rubin: Eat "the Maker's protein," "the Maker's carbohydrates," "the Maker's fiber,"[10] etc., and you
will get long life and health. Rather than bringing us the good news
of Jesus Christ's death on the cross and God's promises of deliverance
from sin, Rubin reads the Bible to bring us good news about our GI
tracts and promises that we will have strong teeth and lean bodies.

This religion of culinary salvation was condemned by Paul in his
letter to Timothy, where he says that those who require "abstinence
from foods that God created to be received with thanksgiving" are
devoting themselves to the "teachings of demons" (1 Timothy 4:1-3).

What's amazing is that while Christians are busy using borrowed
biblical language to justify our attempts to overthrow death (when
death, in case we missed the memo, has already been thrown over),
the world is perfectly open about its desperate agenda. They know
that eating food is a religious act, and they know that avoiding food
is religious as well.

Michelle Allison writes for *The Atlantic*:

> At a fundamental level, people may feel a twinge of guilt
> for having a body, taking up space, and having appe-
> tites that devour the living things around us. They may
> crave expiation of this guilt, and culture provides not
> only the means to achieve plentiful material comfort,
> but also ways to sacrifice part of that comfort to achieve
> redemption. It is not enough for wellness gurus to sim-
> ply amass the riches of health, beauty, and status—they
> must also deny themselves sugar, grains, and flesh. They
> must pay...
>
> This is why arguments about diet get so vicious, so
> quickly. You are not merely disputing facts, you are pit-
> ting your wild gamble to avoid death against someone
> else's. You are poking at their life raft. But if their diet

proves to be the One True Diet, yours must not be. If they are right, you are wrong. This is why diet culture seems so religious. People adhere to a dietary faith in the hope they will be saved. That if they're good enough, pure enough in their eating, they can keep illness and mortality at bay. And the pursuit of life everlasting always requires a leap of faith.[11]

Essayist Mary Eberstadt has observed that our grandmothers had a moral system in which illicit sexuality was outlawed, but women fed their children out of a can without feeling a moment of guilt. This system has been turned on its head in the twenty-first century. Now, a typical 30-year-old woman will use phrases like, "I *should* be juicing more," "I've been so *bad* today," and "I feel so *guilty* for not buying the organic beef." Today's woman now finds her grandmother's sexual attitudes to be outdated and overly moralistic. But in the vacuum of moral boundaries left after the sexual revolution, Eberstadt observes, the human urge to draw up regulations has been transferred to eating.[12] And to underscore the relationship between the pleasures of food and sex, we have the emergence of terms like "food porn."[13]

We also spread moral ideas about food with the vigor of an evangelist, believing that others *ought* to eat the way that we do. Allison observed this as well:

> [Dieting] is a sort of immortality ritual, and rituals must be performed socially. Clean eating rarely, if ever, occurs in secret. If you haven't evangelized about it, joined a movement around it, or been praised publicly for it, have you truly cleansed?[14]

Her words call to mind the somber-faced, fasting Pharisee, exercising his religion in public to be seen by men. Listen for the deeply evangelistic undertones of this exhortation from the blog of vegan content creator Jordan Younger:

> So whether you're into the celery juice hype or not...I am here to tell you: it has worked for countless people around the world, and I trust the Medical Medium wholeheartedly. I haven't stuck with it rigidly enough yet but I am now on Day 2 and I cannot wait to share the benefits with you once I stick with it for a while.[15]

She is an evangelist, with good news to share. She's like another woman at the well, except instead of going home to tell all her friends about a man who offered her living water (John 4:1-42), she is excitedly telling her followers the good news of living celery juice.

Too Much Freedom?

Our worldly attitudes about food flower from the ascetic's underlying assumption—that God is as stingy as we are. Asceticism is being "too proud to enjoy the enjoyable," according to J.I. Packer.[16] It's just legalism, wearing a particularly binding dress. And legalism, as observed by Knute Larson, only "enslaves people to joyless toil." It "lead[s] people down a path of grinding effort, at the end of which there is no God—only insecurities, mental anguish, and more labor."[17]

Perhaps we're more comfortable with mental anguish and labor than with the freedom to walk by the Spirit in enjoying good gifts of physical pleasure. Many of us, depending on the particular lean in our hearts, are simply uncomfortable with the idea of God liking *things*, of God offering us pleasure in *things*. We're uncomfortable with *matter*.

Christian writers like Doug Ponder and Douglas Wilson[18] have observed that God cares how you eat, but he doesn't care what you eat. With perhaps some qualifications that we'll find in other chapters, I think this claim is well supported in Scripture:

> "Food will not commend us to God. We are no worse off if we do not eat, and no better off if we do" (1 Corinthians 8:8).

> "For everything created by God is good, and nothing is to be rejected if it is received with thanksgiving, for it is made holy by the word of God and prayer" (1 Timothy 4:4-5).

> "Whenever you enter a town and they receive you, eat what is set before you" (Luke 10:8).

> "Eat whatever is sold in the meat market without raising any question on the ground of conscience. For 'the earth is the Lord's, and the fullness thereof.' If one of the unbelievers invites you to dinner and you are disposed to go, eat whatever is set before you" (1 Corinthians 10:25-27).

> "Thus [Jesus] declared all foods clean" (Mark 7:19).

> And, last but not least, Peter's epiphany: "Do not call anything impure that God has made clean" (Acts 10:15 KJV).

Perhaps we're just uncomfortable with all this freedom. Furthermore, as we'll address in other chapters, there are complications. We're living in a time of excess. The table as it has been historically used is slipping away, replaced by the couch, the car, and the computer desk. We can't stop eating, and we know that this is a problem. Obviously, our asceticism isn't flowering out of some deep and abiding satisfaction in our culinary habits. If we were happy with the way things were going, would we be so driven to erect the food laws? Obviously, gluttony is a problem for us. You might be thinking, *What then? Are we to turn ourselves over to gluttony?*

This not my proposal. Asceticism rightly fears gluttony; it fears the hostile takeover of the senses. And material worship is no more Christian than asceticism. Even given my feelings about a free conscience, I recognize that we all have consciences tuned to a different key. I find myself uncomfortable when I say this: *If someone eats nothing but McDonald's and high fructose corn syrup, they are not morally wrong in doing so. They are free to eat what their consciences tell them.*

But if I follow my discomfort to its logical end, I find that I'm not sure where it ends: *If someone eats tons of corn syrup every day of their lives, they're wrong.* This could lead to: *If someone eats fast food, they're wrong. If someone eats white bread, they're wrong. Wheat bread. Unsprouted bread. If someone eats sugar, honey, carbohydrates of any kind, meat, dairy...* There is a continuum, and the thing is, we live in such a religiously charged diet culture that there are people who would affirm every one of the statements I just made. There are some who would be uncomfortable exonerating moms who allow their children to consume gluten.

So if I can't allow someone to imbue gluten or meat with moral significance, then can I be allowed to declare McDonald's food unclean? McDonald's once a week? Thrice a week? Every day? Can't we make some kind of value judgment here? Are we supposed to turn ourselves into nutritional agnostics for the sake of a free conscience? What about ethical questions to do with animal cruelty, the environment, and human labor? Are we to ignore those?

No. We all know slippery-slope arguments are lazy. So I propose to approach these questions from another direction. The way I want to establish helpful moral guidelines is to focus on something besides the *substance* of what we eat. Instead, I want to turn our attention to the *way* that we eat. Rather than trying to establish what substances are so bad they just need to be off the table (fast food, preservatives, CAFO meat, GMO grains, etc.), we should redirect our focus, developing virtues that should govern our eating (thanksgiving, temperance, responsibility, and generosity to replace fear, gluttony, apathy, and grabbiness). Through this theological framework, we should be able to tiptoe our way into a theology that addresses the frequency of McDonald's visits.

Unfortunately, for a lot of us, this is not as easy as picking which parts of the food pyramid we're allowed to eat from. We'll have to continue our conversation to get a fuller picture of what the Christian life proposes to do about food.

And so we shall.

FOOD FOR THOUGHT

Discuss

- How many diets have you been on in the last five years? How have these blessed your life, and how have they detracted from your life?

- Having read about the four poles in the Introduction, can you guess which of the four you tend to be drawn to? Or is it a combination of several?

- Do you worry about what would happen if you let go of the food rules you're currently following?

Practice

- Think of a meal that you could eat with pleasure, regardless of whether it fits into the guidelines you have most recently followed. Cook or buy this meal and enjoy it, with company if possible. Eat until you're full, and then stop. Ask yourself whether this meal was good for the soul.

- Pray for help identifying the ditches you yourself are most prone to fall into around food. Specifically, pray for the Holy Spirit's help in identifying areas where you have allowed the ascetic's worldview ("God is as stingy as we are") to infiltrate your heart.

- Pray for guidance as you seek to enjoy God's good gifts without turning them into idols.

Read

- Peruse *A History of Food* by Maguelonne Toussaint-Samat, or any other fairly accessible book by a food historian. It's helpful and fascinating to remember how people have lived and eaten for most of history, in contrast to the ways we live and eat today. We need help dispelling romantic ideas about how much better things were "back then."

- Read *Consumed* by Michelle Stacey for a 1990s perspective on diet culture in America.

CHAPTER 2

Sometimes I Eat the Whole Pint

GLUTTONY AT THE TABLE

In their greed and solicitude, the gluttons seem absolutely to sweep the world with a drag-net to gratify their luxurious tastes. These gluttons, surrounded with the sound of hissing frying-pans, and wearing their whole life away at the pestle and mortar, cling to matter like fire. More than that, they emasculate plain food, namely bread, by straining off the nourishing part of the grain.

—CLEMENT OF ALEXANDRIA[1]

From Memory: 2008

I stand behind a glass counter at 10:45 a.m. There are streaks of sugar glaze on my apron and arms. The smell of grease and dough permeates the shop, my hair, my clothing. On trays under the glass are just the pickings—a few plain cakes, a full tray of plain glazed next to a dwindling tray of blueberry, a small pile of chocolate holes.

There is still an assortment of muffins, though, and the bagels are holding up well. The "kolaches," as they are called in an American donut shop, are just large pigs in a blanket—six-inch sausages wrapped in our house biscuit dough and cheese. This donut shop may be the oldest in Nashville, and it is one of the best. Just basic, old-fashioned donuts (no cronut nonsense in those days) and some other baked goods, all available for about a buck apiece.

I've been at work behind the counter since 4:45 a.m., and I am full and miserable. This job is dangerous for me, and here's why: We're allowed to eat whatever we want while on duty. This means that I pop a few holes when I get in to work, toast a bagel and spread it heavy with honey-almond cream cheese at 10:00 a.m., and begin a slow descent into carbohydrate madness from that point on. During this particularly dangerous season, the donut shop also has a soft-serve machine behind the counter with waffle cones. At 10:45 a.m., when I'm about to get off, I can sometimes convince myself it's socially acceptable to be eating a first cone of the day.

When I finish my shift, I hastily assemble a to-go bag ("for my roommates") and make off with a muffin, two cake donuts, an apple fritter, and a handful of holes. I am embarrassed grabbing them not because of the volume in the bag, but because I feel certain that anyone looking at me can see how uncomfortably full I already am and can guess that this bag will never last long enough for my roommates to see it.

In fact, I already know what I will do. I will drive home, unhappily, lock myself in an empty apartment, eat the remainder of what is in the bag, and relieve myself of the fullness by throwing up.

The other thing I know for sure is that I won't be capable of enjoying a single bite of what's in this bag. Enjoyment was reserved for the morning donut holes, and perhaps the first three bites of the bagel or the cone. In fact, nothing else that I eat today will be enjoyable. Everything that goes into my mouth will be mindlessly, mirthlessly downed—with neither hunger nor community in mind. It will invariably be from a list of "bad carbs" that is always in my head, the list to choose from when I'm already having a "bad day."

This kind of a day starts with a cheerful feeling of emptiness and promise, a party feeling of treating myself for hard work. But lately, it always ends with an isolated, shameful trip to the bathroom. And perhaps another round.

I'll just have to start over tomorrow.

The Fool's "Again, Again"

Gluttony is the fool's impulse to say "again, again" when it is not time for "again." The glutton's heart wants pleasure, and in unlimited amounts. The glutton cannot bear to be human and to have only one mouth, one nose, one pair of eyes, and one stomach with which to enjoy only one breakfast, one lunch, and one supper a day.

Because gluttony is a sin of desire run amok, it's common for us to think that we're gluttonous because we like food too much. Food is too good, we think, and we love it too well—this is why we turn it into an idol. But I contend that gluttony is not a problem of excessive pleasure. It's a problem of pleasure that never reaches its fulfillment.

This is often the case with idolatry. Things we worship become bitter or bland to our taste when we do them up in stone and try to make them last forever. So, we continue to bow before them longer and longer. We worship harder, thinking the first enjoyment will return, but it doesn't. In the end, everything loses its taste—the Creator that we discarded in our reach for created things, and then the created things as well. We could have enjoyed the food both for its own sake, because it is good, and for the sake of the Creator, who made the food as an exposition of his bountiful nature. Instead, we become incapable of enjoying either.

At the beginning of the idolatry process, we think that we love our idols because they are too strong—stronger than the taste of their Creator. (If we could only see him, touch him, taste him! Then we wouldn't need to carve these idols for ourselves!) But when we capitulate to "again, again," we never learn a sweeter truth: *Created things become more potent to us, not less, when loved for the sake of the One who made them. This is part of the Creator's kindness.* In order to taste things fully, we have to know the One who made them, and we have to look to him for direction in our enjoyment. The God who gave limits to the tides has also given limits to our stomachs. These things are good, very good. We can eat with thanksgiving and get the full spectrum of what a meal has to offer, or we can dive our heads into a shallow bowl of pleasure, demanding repetition.

We can savor things for what they are. But in order to enrich our experience, we must ground this love for the things created in a love for the One who created them.[2] When food is used as a shaft of glory that we "look along"[3] in order to see God more clearly—food becomes more sweet, more savory, more strong, more enjoyable.

My gluttony feels nothing like this fully engaged kind of eating. My gluttony is not even the childlike "again and again" that Chesterton attributes to God when God keeps on creating daisies (because he just likes them).[4] Mine is the fool's "again and again" that didn't even really enjoy the first bite, and so keeps eating more and more in an effort to get the missing pleasure that I sense is available but have no capacity to enjoy.

God's "again, again" is an appetite that sees each daisy and delights fully in it. God can appreciate the daisyness of a daisy without destroying that daisyness—even while he continues to create and enjoy millions of them. His capacity for enjoyment is infinitely greater than ours. And our capacity for enjoyment always contracts when we practice idolatry. Rather than a growing appreciation for the created goods that we are consuming—an apple pie, a melon, a bag of Doritos—idolatry produces a shrinking and increasingly unthinking attitude toward the created good.

Michael Pollan describes the experience with junk food that

most of us have had—an experience that propels us toward further gluttony or toward restriction:

> What is it about fast food? Not only is it served in a flash, but more often than not it's eaten that way too: We finished our meal in under ten minutes. Since we were in the convertible and the sun was shining, I can't blame the McDonald's ambiance. Perhaps the reason you eat food this quickly is because it doesn't bear savoring. The more you concentrate on how it tastes, the less like anything it tastes. I said before that McDonald's serves as a kind of comfort food, but after a few bites I'm more inclined to think they're selling something more schematic than that—something more like a signifier of comfort food. So you eat more and eat more quickly, hoping somehow to catch up to the original idea of a cheeseburger or French fry as it retreats over the horizon. And so it goes, bite after bite, until you feel not satisfied exactly, but simply, regrettably, full.[5]

We begin to forget what it was like to enjoy the things as they were meant to be enjoyed. Perhaps there was a moment when we had apple pie for the first time, or when we had the first bite of this particular apple pie, when we tasted the flavor of cinnamon in the crust as it played against the texture of the cooked apples, but that moment was soon overtaken. So we continued until we were sick, eating a second and a third piece. Vaguely, we knew that the pie was a created good and meant to be very enjoyable, but when the enjoyment began to dull, our fool's "again, again" said we should continue to pursue it until it delivered the goods promised.

Then, when the goods delivered a sick stomach, we spoke of pie with disgust. Pie was the problem—*sugar is addictive, you know*! But it didn't occur to us that perhaps it was our ingratitude, our incapacity for enjoyment, and our fool's attitude of demanded repetition that kept us from loving God by enjoying his pie.

Taking the Waves That Come

None of this addresses the question of whether or not to eat a piece of pie when pie is available. I won't tell you whether pie is right for you on a Tuesday night at the women's Bible study (or how to navigate the crucial factors: i.e., whether you are already full, whether the pie was homemade or brought in from Costco, whether there will be ice cream, and whether that ice cream will come from a plastic tub or a Bluebell carton, etc.).

I am only feeling around for a new way of thinking about this familiar spiral into gastronomic discomfort and despair. Perhaps it's not that the pie got ahold of you, but that you never properly got ahold of the pie. It's that, perhaps, you never learned to think of life as waves coming toward you directly from God, waves that you must embrace as they come and then put behind you, readying yourself for the next wave. Waves cannot be repeated at will. Neither can the first bite of pie.

This idea of moments as waves is borrowed from Lewis's novel *Perelandra*. It's from a conversation the main character has with "the Lady," who is the Eve of her own unfallen planet. Here, she comments on the process of accepting a good thing from God's hand:

> "What you have made me see," answered the Lady, "is as plain as the sky, but I never saw it before. Yet it has happened every day. One goes into the forest to pick food and already the thought of one fruit rather than another has grown up in one's mind. Then it may be, one finds a different fruit and not the fruit one thought of. One joy was expected and another is given. But this I had never noticed before—that the very moment of the finding

there is in the mind a kind of thrusting back, or setting aside. The picture of the fruit you have *not* found is still, for a moment, before you. And if you wished—if it were possible to wish—you could keep it there. You could send your soul after the good you had expected, instead of turning it to the good you had got. You could refuse the real good; you could make the real fruit taste insipid by thinking of the other."[6]

The Lady shows us what queenly innocence looks like. She considers everything her Father gives to be a joy, even if it's not the joy she'd originally pictured. In fact, it's a revelation to her to discover that somewhere, somebody might choose to cling to the thing that wasn't given instead of enjoying the fruit in hand. Her simple obedience flows from implicit trust that the Father has only given her joys and will continue to do so, even if some waves are "very swift and great" and may require "all your force to swim into it."[7] She is strong, but her strength is guided and informed by her trust in the Father's giving.

With all of the many difficult things that God ordains in our lives—losses so much greater than a piece of pie—it may seem silly to bring this idea back to food. But if food is where the battleground lies, then there we must fight.

Gluttony gets hung up on the thing that is not given (another first piece of pie) instead of joyfully taking the next wave that God sends (which may be an afternoon work session, a quiet evening at home with the kids, a conversation that will require effort, or a nap). There's always something to go and do next after you eat a piece of pie, and when you resist that next thing in favor of continuing the wave that you liked better, you're seeking to turn back into a wave that has passed. You are clinging to an imaginary piece of fruit instead of riding with thanksgiving the next wave your Father has sent for you.

Tastelessness and Gluttony

I want to expand further on the idea that gluttony is ultimately a kind of tastelessness. It is not the act of attending too closely to the food and enjoying it too much. In fact, gluttony is attending too little to the gift of food and failing to enjoy it.

When my husband and I started dating, our early appointments were for "porch sits." He would come to the house where I was staying, and I would cook him a meal, and we would sit out on the porch and eat it. The retired woman I was staying with would be inside, acting as unofficial chaperone. The view was astonishing: 180 degrees of Tennessee hills from an endless covered porch that felt like it was suspended on air.

One evening as the sun slipped into the trees, we sat eating chicken tenderloin, salad, and potatoes. Justin asked me about my food struggles. Specifically, he asked what he could do to help. I thought for a moment.

"This," I finally answered, gesturing at the view, the supper, and the two rocking chairs we had pulled up to the edge of a rough-hewn, decorative side table where I'd spread the plates and glasses.

"What do you mean?"

"I mean that when I'm having a bad food day, the problem seems to be not too close an association with my food, but that I'm disconnected completely from it. What I don't seem to do on bad food days is cook, or even sit down at a table and eat. I'm in the car, or on the couch, or standing up in front of the pantry or something. There's no thanksgiving; there's little pleasure. For me to cook a meal means I have to spend time on it, think about someone besides myself, and then sit down, give thanks, and treat food like food."

It seems counterintuitive to say that the best way to combat excessive eating is to *eat*, but this has been my experience again and again. Fighting the tastelessness with gratitude and attention has been the basis of my battle against gluttony.

Tastelessness and Dieting

Now—how are gluttony and asceticism connected? In our last chapter, we talked about the strangely religious nature of the food fads. I only briefly touched on the fact that asceticism doesn't spring out of nowhere. Asceticism is almost always a reaction of fear. It's a reaction of fear after experiencing a loss of control.

When you lose your self-control to gluttony—every so often, or for many years—you begin to develop real fear. *Will I ever stop?* you wonder. What could be more natural than attempting to tamp down the impulses of your flesh by setting up rules? And when these rules don't work, what could be more natural than starting over, trying again with new rules, stricter ones? When your body begins to change, to respond to all that fleshly indulgence by producing more flesh, what could be more natural than to panic and start asking around for more rules you've never heard of?

Paul recorded this frustrating cyclical relationship with the law in Romans 7: "I was once alive apart from the law, but when the commandment came, sin came alive and I died. The very commandment that promised life proved to be death to me. For sin, seizing an opportunity through the commandment, deceived me and through it killed me" (7:9-11).

Here he's talking not about man-made religion but about the true law of God. And even this perfect law proved to be death for him. Sin reacts to the law like a mule, bucking and pawing. Later in the passage, Paul reflects on the frustration of being a fallen man: "For I do not understand my own actions. For I do not do what I want, but I do the very thing I hate" (Romans 7:15).

This is what it feels like to be sold as slaves to the passion for food.

We don't understand our own actions. We do the very thing we hate. We know that Scripture itself frowns on what we do. "Be not among drunkards," says the writer of Proverbs, "or among gluttonous eaters of meat. For the drunkard and the glutton will come to poverty, and slumber will clothe them with rags" (23:20-21).

Knowing this to be true, our first impulse is to rectify the problem with the law. We attempt to rein in our bodies with rules that disconnect us from taste by artificially connecting us to terms like *glycemic index* and *cholesterol*. But these invented rules kill the very God-given instincts that might have helped us.

Even though he was writing in the 1960s when the term *calorie* was new to public use, Robert Capon writes about dieting and the loss of taste in ways that still ring true:

> In fact, of course, the insane distinction of fattening/dietetic...fastens its attention, not on food, but on little invisible spooks called calories...Consequently, the dieter has no way of distinguishing good food from bad. Take éclairs, for example. The world is full of them, mostly awful. Any true eater...will be able to give you an accurate judgment as to which of them are worth meeting and which should be avoided. The dieter, however, has lost all criteria for judgment. That éclairs are fattening is his sole piece of information. If he is in a mood to diet, he will pass up the best éclair in the world without even a backward look; if he is in a mood to eat, he will devour a corner-bakery, cardboard-and-cornstarch monstrosity as if it were something out of Brillat-Savarin. He is a man who, for all practical purposes, has lost his taste. He will choose tough steak in the presence of elegant stew, and canned stringed beans when he might have dined on mashed parsnips drenched in butter. All because he has fabricated a set of distinctions which has nothing to do with the subject.[8]

Isn't this just the most familiar description of what it's like to be on a diet? Avoid carbs, and you find that suddenly stale French bread is attractive to you—just because you're not supposed to eat it. Avoid sugar, and you find yourself willing to eat ice cream from a plastic bucket. Avoid meat, and soon you won't know the difference between a tender piece of flank steak and a McNugget. Or if you know the difference, the difference will cease to be a factor in your decision-making. You'll avoid the best on a "good day," and devour the worst on a "bad day." Do this for long enough—months, years, a lifetime—and eventually, you'll be arguing that sugar-free chocolate protein powder tastes just as good as honest-to-goodness chocolate.

Pleasure in food comes from a host of sources: the sight of the food, the smell of the food, the knowledge you have of that food's nutritional properties, and the way the food makes you feel physically when you have eaten it, as well as the texture and taste of the food. It's all right to allow nutritional benefits of food to lead you to enjoy that food more, to choose it over something else. For instance, I eat and enjoy steel-cut oats. Would I eat them if they weren't good for me? Probably not. But the knowledge that they are better for me than most cereals calls my attention to them, allowing me to sit down and eat them with relish and enjoyment. I've found that my tastes tend to expand to include new things I try just because they're healthy. Same goes for vegetables—would I choose to fill plates with veggies if I didn't know they were going to be of long-term benefit to me and my family? Maybe, maybe not. But the fact remains that I eat and love them and can savor each bite of them if they're cooked right. They deserve their place on my table, and they enhance my enjoyment of other ingredients.

I still think nutritional value shouldn't be your only reason for eating something you hate, particularly when it's a trendy ingredient. Some of this stuff—especially the stuff that makes headlines—may be declared out of favor again in a few years. How would you feel if you had been eating—to pick a crazy example for effect—sugary, fat-free, packaged diet food for a decade (let's say it was the '90s), and you hated it all the while, and then one day the expert opinion changed, and you were told you'd been eating something you hated for a decade, and it wasn't even making you thinner—then what? Don't rely too heavily on breaking news about what's good for you. Some things never change. Vegetables, for instance, have always been good for you and always will be. Eat them. Find ways to cook them so that you can appreciate each of them in their natural glory.

Allow the nutritional value of food to contribute its overall enjoyment for you. There's a reason God gave them so many different flavors! It's because they're also full of many different invisible properties that, come to find out, he ordained to contribute various things to the human body. Praise him from whom all blessings flow, and learn to glaze carrots.

Sin and Pleasure

The gluttonous person is sinning. We know this to be true, even if, as Jonathan Edwards observes, "Persons very often deal very perversely in pretending that the sins in which they live are not known sins."[9] We may go days, weeks, or months participating in gluttony, not admitting to ourselves that we are actively pursuing sin. It is easy, with this one, to pretend that the problem is somehow undiagnosed, not a "known sin."

But Scripture gives clarifying instruction:

> Do you not know that your body is a temple of the Holy Spirit within you, whom you have from God? You are not your own. For you were bought at a price. So glorify God in your body (1 Corinthians 6:19-20).

"All things are lawful for me," but not all things are helpful. "All things are lawful for me," but I will not be dominated by anything. "Food is meant for the stomach and the stomach for food"—and God will destroy both one and the other. The body is not meant for sexual immorality, but for the Lord, and the Lord for the body (1 Corinthians 6:12-13).

In these passages about sexual immorality, we find clear application to our other bodily passions. Our bodies are not our own. All things may be lawful, but not all things are helpful. We must not be dominated by anything. The body is not meant for sexual immorality (or miserable overeating), but for the Lord. We were bought with a price; therefore, we should glorify God in our bodies.

Conviction sets in as we read these verses. So we can't be gluttons, but we can't be ascetics either? Then how can we address the gluttony? It will continue until it's addressed—that much we know. The appetites are alive and well. The habits are well established.

Michelle Stacey talks about American food obsession from her vantage point in the '90s, and hints at a solution that I want to take to the sanctified level of Christian worship:

> Americans are not eating right. Our many contortions in the face of our food—self-denial, fear, obsessiveness, hope for magical salvation—all spring from attempts to redress that same wrong. But the true cure for our dietary sins may lie in an almost opposite direction to that prescribed by the nutrition cognoscenti: not in claiming more control, but less; not in taking power away from food, but giving it back; not in fear of death, but in love of life. Somewhere in the ancient love of food and its rituals lies rationality and reverence for natural things and a balanced sense of how much is too

much—colored by scientific knowledge, but not ruled by it.[10]

She continues:

> One central, and rather ironic, problem with the food paranoids' answer to this bad eating is that it is often based on some of the very proclivities that have helped lead to an impoverished cuisine: a disregard for pleasure, and even more basically, a disrespect for the power and the symbolism of food. Even when we went about consciously changing something for the better, the underlying disrespect for food remained the same. For example, one of the replacements for the admittedly unhealthy American breakfast of eggs, bacon, sausage, and buttered toast has been the Carnation Instant Breakfast drink, an early symbol of techno-foods, whose recent advertising tag line is: "Because life doesn't stop for breakfast." The question that is begged here is, Why not? Maybe it should. Certainly it should stop for dinner.[11]

Stacey's vision to reconnect with a "love of life" is much to be preferred to the obsession and disconnect she was seeing in 1995. But our vision as Christians should be so much greater. We should be filled with gratitude for our food: not gratitude to "natural things" but gratitude to the overflowing, fertile God of plenty and pleasure, the God who promises us an eternal feast as a picture of the heaven that awaits (Matthew 22:1-14; Isaiah 25:6; Song of Solomon 2:4). We should be checked and balanced in our enjoyments, not by "rationality" but by the self-control that is promised as the fruit of the Holy Spirit (Galatians 5:22-23). We should learn, with Paul in 1 Corinthians 6, not to be dominated by anything because of our deep joy in glorifying God in our bodies.

The true answer to gluttony has much more in common with

feasting than with dieting. It has to do with worship, gratitude, and generosity. It is becoming more and more a child who receives, and less and less a parent who withholds (from ourselves and those around us). It is sitting quietly and with full presence of mind, glorying in tastes that were created by a good God, instead of fearing and distrusting tastes that were made *too* good by a good God. The answer to gluttony is knowing when enough is enough, learning the feel of a wave passing, and growing in the wisdom that looks to the next wave from God with satisfaction, contentment, and readiness.

FOOD FOR THOUGHT

Discuss

- In this chapter, gluttony was described as the fool's "again, again." Have you had the experience of returning to food again and again and finding that satisfaction didn't come?

- Discuss the idea that God's providence is like a wave that comes and then passes, followed by a different wave. What are some of the waves that you avoid swimming into after you're done eating? Tasks or unpleasant parts of your day that lead you to try to turn back into the wave of food after a meal should be over?

- Have you ever tried to control uncontrolled eating by setting up new and increasingly restrictive food rules?

Practice

- For one week, give yourself only one guideline for eating: Sit down at a table for everything you consume this week. Give thanks for each meal, and pay attention to it to the degree that you're able.

- Pray for the Holy Spirit's conviction this week for those occasions when you sin by worshiping food, eating far past the point of enjoyment, or using the food to avoid responsibilities he's given you. Confess this sin to the Lord as it comes, and move on.

Read

- Read *Perelandra* by C.S. Lewis for its fascinating take on repetition of pleasure (he compares another bite of especially sweet alien fruit to a request for an orchestra to play the symphony over again in the same day).[12] This is also worth reading for its imaginative retelling of Eve's temptation on another planet.

CHAPTER 3

You Aren't Eating Maca Root?

SNOBBERY AT THE TABLE

A new report by the Bible Scholars of America found that Adam and Eve were actually punished for eating the forbidden fruit in the Garden of Eden because the fruit was genetically modified.

—BABYLON BEE

From Memory: 1995

I am seven years old. I am sitting at a 12-foot, green-legged farm table with a bowl of Honeycomb cereal in front of me. The yellow color of the cereal fills my vision, and my heart is singing. I spoon four honeycombs into one bite and bring it to my mouth, marveling at the perfect hexagonal shape of each piece. How do they get them all to look the same? Six perfect holes, each another opportunity for milk to be trapped.

The bite in my mouth is sweet. It is satisfyingly spongy—the milk in those holes and the milk that has been sopped up by the dry, foamy bulk of each piece is now being extracted by my baby molars. There is a crunch too, provided by the exterior glaze of something that is purportedly honey but probably has a more direct relationship with corn syrup.

My three sisters sit at the table as well, each crunching their way through a first or second bowl. Two more enormous Honeycomb boxes are on the kitchen counter—is this really happening?

This dream-turned-reality has come upon us so quickly, and without even a hint of a lobby. Driving home like normal from the store, Papa suddenly made an announcement: We've purchased three boxes of Honeycomb and, when we get back to the farmhouse, we're allowed to eat it for supper. As much as we want, for supper. Do we have to mix it? No, no mixing. Just Honeycomb, for supper.

Usually we have to mix any cereal that falls into the category of "sugary" (Frosted Shredded Wheat, honey-nut anything, Raisin Bran) with a benign filler (Cheerios, Corn Flakes, plain Shredded Wheat). This has been my mother's attempt to stem the tide of sugar rushes for years.

Except, for some reason, on this night. On this night, the rules don't apply. On this night, Papa is sitting there refilling his bowl and giggling with the rest of us. I sit in the chair and close my eyes with pleasure. It is too much. For some reason, this will be one of the most memorable meals of my life.

Ungraciously Paleo

I was sitting in a Mexican restaurant recently, and at the next table I overheard one of the funniest orders I've ever witnessed. A young man was sitting with four or five of his peers, and a polite waitress attended them.

"Okay, so I'm Paleo," the young man began. He looked around at his friends and shrugged. "I've been Paleo ever since I read the book...it's so much better for you." The waitress listened patiently. He turned back to her with the air of a man who is speaking words of eternal significance.

"So I want to know what is in your corn tortilla chips. Are they low carb? Because they need to be...if they're not low carb they're probably not Paleo. And what about your beef enchiladas—are they Paleo? I've only been Paleo for a little while now, so I haven't been in a Mexican restaurant since. I bet it's hard to be Paleo at a Mexican restaurant. So Paleo means that you only eat things you can basically kill or dig up...do you have any dishes that are pretty much just meat and maybe nuts? I think it would be Paleo to eat like the oil on the meat but maybe not if there's cheese on it..."

Slowly, the truth was becoming clear to everyone at the table: This young man was Paleo.

"Paleo?" said the waitress. There was more meaning packed into this one word and the expression on her face than in some sermons I've heard.

"Yes, Paleo. Have you heard of it?" He continued ordering for probably two more minutes. His friends squirmed.

The absurd caricature presented by the young man in the Mexican restaurant is funny because most of the people we know are too self-aware to repeat the word *Paleo* 12 times while ordering at a Mexican restaurant. But his behavior is also uncomfortably familiar—most of us have followed diets, and most of us have spent time and effort explaining those diets to someone else in a setting like this one. Most of us have been inconvenienced by our diets, and who knows? It's at least possible that we have inconvenienced friends and family members.

For a book written more than 50 years ago, *The Screwtape Letters* by C.S. Lewis offers a terribly relevant diagnosis of our finicky food behavior. Here, the demon Screwtape describes an older woman's food fussiness with a word that would shock her: *gluttony*.

She would be astonished—one day, I hope will be—to

learn that her whole life is enslaved to this kind of sensuality, which is quite concealed from her by the fact that the quantities involved are small. But what do quantities matter, provided we can use a human belly and palate to produce querulousness, impatience, uncharitableness, and self-concern? Glubose has this old woman well in hand. She is a positive terror to hostesses and servants.[1]

What does this lady's gluttony look like? It's not what you'd expect. She's a small British woman who doesn't eat much. But Screwtape says the demons have accomplished great things in Europe by concentrating their efforts on "the gluttony of Delicacy, not on the gluttony of Excess." So they've produced people like this woman:

> She is always turning from what has been offered her to say with a demure little sigh and a smile "Oh please, please...*all* I want is a cup of tea, weak but not too weak, and the teeniest weeniest bit of really crisp toast." You see? Because what she wants is smaller and less costly than what has been set before her, she never recognizes as gluttony her determination to get what she wants, however troublesome it may be to others.[2]

If you want to recognize this woman in present-day America, just substitute some of her favorite phrases for others: "Is there sugar in this muffin?" "Oh, I'm all right—thanks for making that—but I'll just have a cup of coffee. I'm trying to avoid dairy." "I'm sorry, ma'am, but this latte is just a tad too cold. Could you have them make another and bring it? And could I just have some agave nectar for the table?"

The gluttony of delicacy may be most damaging to the soul of the person who practices it, but it also affects the lives of others. I think of snobbery as a social outworking of some of the very food sins we've already discussed. Many of the women who show this kind of behavior in other people's homes or in restaurants aren't doing it because it's fun. They're doing it because they're afraid. They're doing it because they've been on the twin treadmills of asceticism and gluttony for so long that they don't recognize basic social graces anymore.

Several times, I've seen a Christian woman show up at someone's house for supper with her own food in Tupperware. Not something she brought to contribute to the meal, but something she brought to eat all by herself—something that fits into the rigid walls of her diet. Once or twice, it was a woman who had a food allergy, who brought her own food as a gracious way of relieving the hostess from the responsibility of navigating that allergy. But usually, it was just a woman who'd recently given up processed flour or sugar or dairy or meat or *fill in the blank*, and it was important enough to her that she couldn't bring herself to trust what was served at the table.

I find these situations embarrassing. I am embarrassed for the woman—a grown person who was presumably taught good manners as a child—who has forgotten her manners. But I'm also embarrassed by the idea that no one even raises an eyebrow because hey, we're probably starting a cleanse tomorrow ourselves. We're impressed with her dedication! The madness is so ubiquitous that we can't even recognize madness anymore.

Kindness as a guest means that where food allergies don't make it impossible, we should be willing to eat what our hosts have taken the trouble to make for us. In our culture, it doesn't mean we have to burp loudly at the table to express our appreciation (as in some areas of South Asia). But regardless of cultural context, we know this much: When a host makes food, she wants the food to be eaten.

On the flip side, the loving thing to do as a host is to make food with your guests in mind. My mother is a wonderful example of the

selfless host. She herself has been a vegan for several years, but when
her adult children and their families show up for supper, she pulls
out all the stops for them: gorgeous roasts, luscious desserts featuring quality ice cream, and expertly turned out cream pastas regularly grace her table.

Personally, I always ask guests before they come if they have
dietary restrictions. My opinion of the diet is immaterial; if they
mention the diet, I make sure there will be food they can eat. And, of
course, all of this requires wisdom, nuance, and love. There's a range
of behavior here, and a wide range of motives for exceptional eating. Perhaps you're a professional athlete. Perhaps you're pregnant
or nursing. Perhaps you're diabetic or have a serious food allergy.
Maybe you just want a smaller piece of cake. The takeaway here isn't
"Never under any circumstances make requests to suit your dietary
needs or preferences." The takeaway here is this: "Let love be genuine. Abhor what is evil; hold fast to what is good...Contribute to the
needs of the saints and seek to show hospitality" (Romans 12:9,13).

The table fellowship of the church is at stake here in these small
things. Our witness outside the church is at stake. Whether we are
guests or hosts, we should be known as gracious people who are quick
to bend in deference to others. One of the most pleasurable and effective tools we have for connecting with believers and unbelievers—
fellowship over food—is endangered when we allow ourselves to
become fussy eaters. We can't focus on the ministry that takes place
around the table—ministry to individuals with needs that extend
far beyond fear of sugar—when we're intent on flourishing the word
Paleo to anyone who will listen.

Food snobbery isn't just a silly social gaffe. It's an indulgence of
the flesh that may have far-reaching consequences to the spiritual
lives of ourselves and others.

Consumer-Driven Snobbery

Whole Foods is a delicious place to be. And the only one in Franklin, Tennessee, is right around the corner from my parents' house. I sometimes take little pilgrimages over there while my girls are napping, just to walk around and eat the cheese samples.

Walk in the door and you are blasted by the cool air of the produce section. Apples are piled high in perfect symmetry, each individual piece of fruit flawless and valued at twice the price of an apple from my home grocery store. Oranges, mangos, pears, and cherries create nearby pillars of symmetry and color. Along one wall, any green leafy vegetable you can think of is available to be bunched, weighed, and carried home. Along another wall, there are Venti-sized plastic containers full of every combination of chopped gourd and root vegetable you could dream up.

Moving toward the "catch of the day" sign in the back that looks like it was mounted on reclaimed barn wood, you pass a juice-your-own orange station and a row of grind-your-own nut butter machines. Chia, toasted and raw hemp, brown and gold flaxseeds, pumpkin seeds, and black or white sesame seeds are all on tap for bulk purchases. On the back wall, there are smoked meats and a large assortment of cheeses, and more organic dairy products than you can shake an udder at.

The other side of the store is perhaps the most enticing, with its puffy loaves of bread, its display of cakes and tarts and cookies, its fragrant salad bar, its rows of local beer, and its cold-pressed juice, smoothie, gelato, and coffee bars.

The thing that you can't see when you walk through this store is the idea-machine that feeds into the whole enterprise. You don't know who the people are that craft the verbiage on the product descriptions. You don't know that executives thousands of miles away sat in a room with a market researcher who explained to him that using the words *organic* and *cage-free* is not enough; that *locally farmed* and *experience-based* are the new standard. Customers want to know what county their beef was raised in.

You may not be able to hear the meetings that take place in Whole Foods headquarters, but you can go online and read articles about Top Ingredient Trends this year. Online, you'll find a near-exact description of the products available on these shelves and in nearby restaurants:

> Trend #1): Flowers in food: Exhibits include the Whole Foods Market™ Lime Mint Elderflower Italian Sparkling Mineral Water; 365 Everyday Value® Lavender Lemon Granola, Lime Mint Elderflower Juice, and Jacobs Farm Organic Edible Flowers
>
> Trend #3): Functional Mushrooms: See the Kettle & Fire Mushroom Chicken Bone Broth; Om Reishi Mushroom Powder; Alaffia Coconut Reishi Chai Shower Gel
>
> Trend #6): Plant-Based Alternatives: See Sophie's Kitchen Vegan Toona; MALK cold-pressed nut milks; Mooala Bananamilk; Forager Cashew Yogurt
>
> Trend #9): Root-to-Stem: This is about using even the stalks of the vegetable; see the "produce butcher" at Whole Foods Market Bryant Park; Melon Seed Agua Fresca; Butternut Squash with Celery Leaves and Orecchiette[3]

These trends are predictable to a point. They trickle down from the front lines of food culture—chefs and food critics make the trend, industry leaders watch and influence trends as they do purchasing and product development for stores like Whole Foods, and eventually, we get products like banana milk, which may or may not ever make it to a place like my local Aldi.

This trend-trickle reminds me of one described in *The Devil*

Wears Prada by the fashion leader and magazine editor Miranda Priestly:

> You think this has nothing to do with you. You go to your closet and you select...I don't know...that lumpy blue sweater, for instance, because you're trying to tell the world that you take yourself too seriously to care about what you put on your back. But what you don't know is that that sweater is not just blue, it's not turquoise. It's not lapis. It's actually cerulean. And you're also blithely unaware of the fact that in 2002, Oscar de la Renta did a collection of cerulean gowns...
>
> And then cerulean quickly showed up in the collections of eight different designers. And then it, uh, filtered down through the department stores and then trickled on down into some tragic Casual Corner where you, no doubt, fished it out of some clearance bin. However, that blue represents millions of dollars and countless jobs and it's sort of comical how you think that you've made a choice that exempts you from the fashion industry when, in fact, you're wearing the sweater that was selected for you by the people in this room.[4]

Miranda Priestly's devastating takedown can help us understand our own food and drink choices a little more clearly. Maybe we don't know much about food. Maybe we do. Maybe we are a cheerful follower of the newest final word on nutrition, or maybe we are cheerfully feeding our children out of the frozen meal section at Save-A-Lot. But whatever we eat, we are largely dependent on other people for our ingredients and our information. We may feel that we're taking charge of our destinies by following a low-inflammation diet, but we are getting our ideas from fallible people. We may feel like we're cultivated and discriminating consumers who only go for the best, but we are probably just choosing items that have been chosen for us—that the great machine of food industry picked out via consumer trials 15 months ago. And there's no problem with this. It's just that we shouldn't forget it.

We're not special because we eat food that Whole Foods thinks people like us will eat this year. It says nothing about our worth as people. It only says something about the skill of the food salesmen and saleswomen. And more power to them—they make that Lime Mint Elderflower Italian Sparkling Mineral Water sound *good*.

I know people who always have to be the first to hear about a new ingredient. They were talking about chia before it infiltrated Walmart; they know that acai berries are tired and boring, and husk cherries are on the way up. It's a silly thing to be snobbish about, but human beings have always been silly about the things they're snobbish about.

Two hundred years ago in Jane Austen's England, people were bragging about family titles and numbers of servants. For thousands of years in India, a clearly demarcated caste system took the guesswork out of social hierarchies. In modern-day China, the newly wealthy take lessons in snobbery from British etiquette expert James Hebbert.[5] Americans, perhaps, maintain a more complicated caste system than some other cultures have. You can brag about almost anything here (education, lack of education, militant parenting, laid-back parenting, ab definition, "fat pride," vacation plans, career milestones, relationship goals, gut bacteria, etc.). But our caste system is every bit as man-made and self-indulgent as the ones used to torment people in nineteenth-century British drawing rooms or in twelfth-century Indian villages.

Christian women shouldn't be silly women. They shouldn't be arrogant women or snobbish women. They shouldn't be women who try to hang their hats on meaningless identity markers. But, of course, Christian women are people too.

This calls to mind another wonderful word from the tempter Screwtape:

> The man who truly and disinterestedly enjoys any one thing in the world, for its own sake, and without caring twopence what other people say about it, is by that very fact forearmed against some of our subtlest modes of attack. You should always try to make the patient abandon the people or food or books he really likes in favor of the "best" people, the "right" food, the "important" books. I have known a human defended from strong temptations to social ambition by a still stronger taste for tripe and onions.[6]

It's not snobbery to enjoy something enjoyable. Snobbery happens when our enjoyment of a good thing comes from the sense that *someone else out there doesn't have it and wishes they did.* Lewis's word about "tripe and onions" above should suggest to us a healthy exercise: Ask yourself what innocent things you like to eat and read and do, and then do them whenever freedom allows. Participate in something you love, but without ensuring that someone sees you do it. For some of us, this will be a challenge in itself—*how to enjoy something if no one sees you enjoying it?*

Dabbling in Allergies

"I led the church in Communion on Sunday with a rice cracker—weird," writes Kevin DeYoung. "It still seems strange that this is my new lot in life. I suppose Celiac should make me long for the wedding supper of the Lamb, but right now it's making me hungry for monkey bread."[7]

DeYoung is a pastor and a theological writer—not the kind of person you'd expect to blog thousands of words about his gluten intolerance. But he did. In 2016, he published a long article detailing the process through which he was diagnosed with celiac disease. He wrote about his former diet (which was bad enough that while reading I wondered how he was able to stay so "crazy busy" all those years), his increasingly life-altering symptoms, and his many rounds of testing. Finally, he was positively, medically diagnosed with celiac disease, which is a verifiable autoimmune disorder in which ingesting gluten damages the smaller intestine.

Why did DeYoung spend this kind of time and effort in publicly announcing and explaining his diagnosis? I have to think part of it was the necessity of explaining to people that his gluten intolerance was the real deal. Because announcing that you were gluten intolerant in 2016 was a little like announcing you were antiwar in 1969. Everybody around you would just nod and say, "Oh yeah, me too."

A doctor told DeYoung, "I have people come in all the time wanting these tests. Everyone thinks they have gluten problems. I never see anyone test positive. You just did."

It must be frustrating, for the people with life-altering symptoms, who spend months in doctors' offices in order to get answers, to be surrounded by others who practice something more along the lines of a casual allergy dabble. People with serious food allergies have to deal with a lot already. Being caught in a sea of on-again, off-again boutique allergy shoppers shouldn't be one of them.

But it is. The gluten-allergy craze is a great example of a food-fear trend that started with a few books and articles, surged in popularity, and seems to have reached the end of its shelf life (pun intended). The strange behavior around wheat that we saw over the last ten years is fantastic comedy material: "Being gluten intolerant used to be limited to people who were actually intolerant of gluten, but with the cutting-edge information I'm sharing with you in this video, you too can be gluten intolerant," JP Sears said in a video called *How to Become Gluten Intolerant*, which was put out at the height of the craze and viewed over ten million times on YouTube.

In the video, Sears sits calmly and delivers the following lines with a breathtaking deadpan:

> Being gluten intolerant is a fantastic opportunity for you to assert your dominance on the lives of everyone around you—which helps improve your life! So if you're ready to have a ravenous appetite for impossible standards and dogmatic feelings of victimization, then let's get started...
>
> Never let anyone's efforts be good enough for you. If you're at a friend's house, and they've gone out of their way and think they've met the DaVinci Code of your gluten-free demands, they're not trying to be friendly— they're trying to overthrow your reign of control and dominance. You can't let this happen. You'll want to play the trump card of another food intolerance that you've never told them about before. This puts you back in the driver's seat.[8]

It may seem like this allergy-dabbling is not a big deal. After all, it affects our social interactions, but it doesn't stop them from happening. The extra meal can be made for those with faux allergies just like it can be made for those with genuine allergies. But to see the spiritual ramifications of making yourself difficult to your friends and waitresses, we return to our gluttonous old British lady:

> The real value of the quiet, unobtrusive work which Glubose has been doing for years on this old woman can be gauged by the way in which her belly now dominates

her whole life. The woman is in what may be called the "All-I-want" state of mind. All she wants is a cup of tea properly made, or an egg properly boiled, or a slice of bread properly toasted. But she never finds any servant or any friend who can do these simple things "properly"— because her "properly" conceals an insatiable demand for the exact, and almost impossible, palatal pleasures which she imagines she remembers from the past; a past described by her as "the days when you could get good servants" but known to us as the days when her senses were more easily pleased and she had pleasures of other kinds which made her less dependent on those of the table. Meanwhile, the daily disappointment produces daily ill temper: cooks give notice and friendships are cooled. If ever the Enemy introduces into her mind a faint suspicion that she is too interested in food, Glubose counters it by suggesting to her that she doesn't mind what she eats herself but "does like to have things nice for her boy." In fact, of course, her greed has been one of the chief sources of his domestic discomfort for years.[9]

All you want, you may think, is to have more energy. All you want is to feel that you are taking control of your health by never touching milk products again. But this all-I-want may become the thing that spiritually dominates your life. It may be that you have a profound theological misunderstanding that turns you into a difficult guest and a difficult customer. It may be that your simple demands for a special plate are just a mask for your spiritual demand to be made much of.

Three Mistakes

There are three theological misunderstandings—three mistakes—that I think contribute to our unkind food behavior in the church.

The social behavior described in this chapter—high-maintenance food orders, bringing your own meal to someone's house without medical cause, or trying to make your friends feel foolish because they've never heard of yacon syrup—doesn't develop out of nowhere. A Christian has to swallow something deeply untrue about God and the world around her before her vision becomes so distorted that this kind of behavior feels natural.

Mistake #1: Being surprised by death and disease in a sin-cursed world

For some, it is a false doctrine built into their explicit theology (i.e., prosperity-gospel teaching that God promises health as part of the atoning work of Christ). But I think that for most of us, it's subconscious. It's part of a system we don't even know is in our hearts, a quid pro quo system we'd like to have with God. According to this system, we hope that if we do everything right, God will ensure that we're energetic and well.

The problem is that we are thinking too little about the fall and too little about what is promised to us in the new heavens and new earth. It's basic unbelief. We know things are broken in this age. We know Christ died to deliver us from sin's curse, and he's coming back to usher in a new age in which "everything sad [is] going to come untrue" (to quote one of our favorite hobbits).[10] But to the degree that we doubt this promise in our hearts—to that exact degree—we will be tempted to cling to dietary promises as a way of defeating death. Our doubt will render us helpless to let go of these dietary promises even when good sense and love of neighbor dictate. We won't be able to talk about anything but food and health with our friends because that's what we'll be thinking about all the time.

I know women who regularly respond to descriptions of health issues with dietary diagnoses. If someone has cancer, they declare that a better diet would have prevented it. If someone has sleep or behavior problems, they know what nutritional deficiencies cause them. And, of course, there's always some truth in the assumption that health and diet are connected in verifiable ways. But I wonder if in our endless discussions of disease prevention, we've forgotten something obvious: We're all dying.

The psalmist reminds us of what we all know in our quiet moments:

> He knows our frame;
> 　he remembers that we are dust.
> As for man, his days are like grass;
> 　he flourishes like a flower of the field;
> for the wind passes over it, and it is gone,
> 　and its place knows it no more (103:14-16).

James warns those of us who would arrogantly assume we have another day on this earth coming to us:

> Come now, you who say, "Today or tomorrow we will go into such and such a town and spend a year there and trade and make a profit"—yet you do not know what tomorrow will bring. What is your life? For you are a mist that appears for a little time and then vanishes. Instead you ought to say, "If the Lord wills, we will live and do this or that." As it is, you boast in your arrogance. All such boasting is evil (James 4:13-16).

If our minds are steeped in Scripture, the slow or (quick) wasting away of flesh is impossible to forget. The Word of God tells us over and over again that this present world is marked by death and decay, and nothing can stop this process except supernatural intervention. The Christian, like everybody else, rightly feels that death is unnatural. But instead of clinging to scientific breakthroughs or

2,000-year-old forgotten herbs, she must cling to the promises of God.

God has pledged the following to us: new bodies, which will allow us to live in a new heavens and a new earth. Jesus has already conquered death, and someday it will be swallowed up forever. But in the meantime, we've been prepared for what's coming, and we don't have to be surprised or shocked by it. As we watch our bodies die, we mourn, but we also rest. Jesus told us this was coming (John 14:1-3; 16:33). He told us not to fear. "So we do not lose heart," says Paul. "Though our outer self is wasting away, our inner self is being renewed day by day" (2 Corinthians 4:16).

Mistake #2: Thinking we can neglect to fill our minds with what is good and true without consequences

This passage about the picky British lady hints for just a second at one of the problems that I think contributes to social food sin. Screwtape says when the lady was younger, "she had pleasures of other kinds which made her less dependent on those of the table." Not anymore. In other words, she is bored. Her mind is a vacuum. She is fixated on getting exactly what she wants at the table because she has nothing else going on up there.

I know very well how all-consuming food concerns can be. I know that during certain seasons of my life, food has taken up most of my waking thoughts. I also know that on a social level, I often open my mouth and say something not because it's the thing I think is most interesting and important to talk about, but because I can't think of anything else to say.

I noticed a few years ago that at church I was always complimenting the other women on their clothing. I don't mean that I just threw out a "Cute dress!" or "What a nice pair of shoes!" now and then. I mean I was leading with this conversational opener on a regular basis. I began to notice a glazed look in the eyes of friends, who could have joyfully discussed many other topics of life, from parenting to work to the sermon we'd both just heard.

But instead, I was regularly catching everybody near me in a cyclical, shallow discussion of where-you-got-that-skirt (because as everybody knows, if someone compliments an article of your clothing, the law of immediate disclosure means you're socially obligated to tell them where you got it). Why was I doing this? I wondered. Then I finally realized why—pure laziness. It was a default mode of conversation to say the first thing that came to my mind, and my mind was often blank of anything but immediate, surface-level observations.

Some women talk about food because they're obsessed and can't sustain thought about anything else. I've been there. But others talk about food just because they don't know what else to talk about. Maybe they aren't experiencing spiritual growth or don't know how to talk about the things of God in a way that feels natural. Maybe they feel out of their depth asking friends to reveal personal and relational struggles. Maybe they are so lost in everyday tasks that they have no vision for the spiritual work God intends them to be about. The fact is, they haven't developed other occupations that could fill the space left if food took a less central role in their hearts and minds and mouths.

Sometimes I think a lot of food-related sin is just space filler, and it rushes in automatically when we aren't busying ourselves with the spiritual and physical work God has given us to do.

The heart issue that leads us to shopping for allergies or bragging about obscure superfoods may be simple idleness. Some of us simply have too much mental space on our hands. We're not about our Father's business—stirring up our own joy, sitting in fellowship with our Lord, sharing his good news with others, speaking words that build up, addressing people's needs—and our idle, empty minds will always find something to occupy them.

Paul exhorted the Philippians to take responsibility for what was in their minds:

> Finally, brothers, whatever is true, whatever is honorable, whatever is just, whatever is pure, whatever is lovely, whatever is commendable, if there is any excellence, if there is anything worthy of praise, think about these things. What you have learned and received and heard and seen in me—practice these things, and the God of peace will be with you (Philippians 4:8-9).

Mistake #3: Thinking we can prioritize health or weight over the good of our neighbor

Paul's letters are full of long passages that explain to us what it looks like to be socially gracious toward our fellow believers. Many of these passages apply directly to table fellowship. Paul was invested in the preservation and promotion of culinary kindness.

As we saw in the chapter on asceticism, Jesus and Paul both took pains to establish dietary freedoms under the new covenant of faith. But Paul also takes pains to explain to believers that no matter what your personal convictions are around food—*you always seek to love and serve the person with whom you're eating.*

He writes to the Romans:

> One person believes he may eat anything, while the weak person eats only vegetables. Let not the one who eats despise the one who abstains, and let not the one who abstains pass judgment on the one who eats, for God has welcomed him. Who are you to pass judgment on the servant of another? It is before his own master

that he stands or falls. And he will be upheld, for the
Lord is able to make him stand (Romans 14:2-4).

We have different convictions. We eat different diets, depending
on our backgrounds, our bodies, our budgets, and our influences.
But we aren't to let that throw us into snobbery. Paul understood the
human heart too well—the one who eats wants to look down on the
weakness of the one who thinks he shouldn't. The one who doesn't eat
wants to look down on the carelessness of the one who thinks he can.

Stop it, says Paul.

> Therefore let us not pass judgment on one another any
> longer, but rather decide never to put a stumbling block
> or hindrance in the way of a brother. I know and am per-
> suaded in the Lord Jesus that nothing is unclean in itself,
> but it is unclean for anyone who thinks it is unclean. For
> if your brother is grieved by what you eat, you are no
> longer walking in love. By what you eat, you are no lon-
> ger walking in love. By what you eat, do not destroy the
> one for whom Christ died (Romans 14:13-15; see also
> 1 Corinthians 8:1-13).

That takes care of the idea that you can look down your nose at
your friend who is under conviction about something like alcohol
or meat given to idols. Paul says that even the freer woman should
rein herself in if she's creating a stumbling block for the weaker sister.

But in 1 Corinthians, he also addresses the flip side, command-
ing those who may lean more on the side of not wanting to eat.
What should they do when they are guests in someone's home and
the person serves them meat that was given to idols?

> Eat whatever is sold in the meat market without rais-
> ing any question on the ground of conscience. For "the
> earth is the Lord's, and the fullness thereof." If one of the

unbelievers invites you to dinner and you are disposed to go, eat whatever is set before you without raising any question on the ground of conscience. But if someone says to you, "This has been offered in sacrifice," then do not eat it, for the sake of the one who informed you, and for the sake of conscience—I do not mean your conscience, but his. For why should my liberty be determined by someone else's conscience? If I partake with thankfulness, why am I denounced because of that for which I give thanks?

So, whether you eat or drink, or whatever you do, do all to the glory of God. Give no offense to Jews or to Greeks or to the church of God, just as I try to please everyone in everything I do, not seeking my own advantage, but that of many, that they may be saved (1 Corinthians 10:25-33).

The key to his whole passage is in 10:24: "Let no one seek his own good, but the good of his neighbor." This is the way we can navigate any position in which we find ourselves. Is someone coming to your house who doesn't partake of several major food groups, and you're convinced that they could probably live quite comfortably some months into the future even if they consumed the spaghetti and meatballs you were planning on serving? Your job isn't to determine whether they're behaving graciously; your job is to graciously serve them. Bend over backward to accommodate. Learn the rules or preferences they list to you, and follow them. Take it as a challenge, a hospitality exercise.

Are you fresh on the no-carb wagon, but you have dinner at the Smiths on Friday night, and you're worried the whole thing will get derailed? Forget about it. The glycemic index will keep. Your fellowship with the Smiths may not, and at any rate, a good night of gracious fellowship will go further toward your health than many months of glycemic holiness is likely to do for you. Go, don't mention the diet, and eat what's set before you. You don't have to eat like a glutton, but neither should you be bringing your own supper in Tupperware. Practice love, and prioritize fellowship over food snobbery.

FOOD FOR THOUGHT

Discuss

- What is the silliest food behavior you've ever participated in? That you've witnessed?

- How do you think food acts as a social marker among the people you know? Do you tend to put people into categories in your mind based on what they eat and where they buy their food?

- What are some practical ways that you could practice love when you're in the position of host? How about when you're the guest?

Practice

- Institute a potluck with your church community. My church is small enough that we are able to do one after services every Sunday. I recognize this is a luxury, and not every church could do this. But it is a great opportunity for learning to eat graciously together.

- Be considerate of those with food allergies. Remember that for those who deal with debilitating reactions to common ingredients, it is harder to eat out, harder to eat in, and harder to buy groceries. Serve them in any way you can.

- Ask those you live with what they'd like for supper this week. Some of us are willing to bend over backward for guests, but we don't know our own spouse's favorite foods.

- Ask yourself whether you are the kind of restaurant patron that wait staff looks forward to seeing. I was a waitress once, and I remember fellow waitresses warning me about a regular, an elderly man who they said was always high maintenance and a poor tipper. I recognized him as the pastor of a local church.

- Buy a nostalgic packaged food from your childhood and eat it for supper. It isn't going to make you any cooler, but isn't it good?

Read

These longer passages of Scripture would be helpful to read in their full context as you seek to examine your social attitudes around food:

- Romans 14
- 1 Corinthians 8
- 1 Corinthians 10

CHAPTER 4

Coq Au Vin ≠ Chicken Nuggets

APATHY AT THE TABLE

"How do you know what you'll like if you won't even try anything?" asked Father.

"Well," said Frances, "there are many different things to eat, and they taste many different ways. But when I have bread and jam I always know what I am getting, and I am always pleased."

—RUSSELL HOBAN, *BREAD AND JAM FOR FRANCES*[1]

From Memory: 2019

I stand in the backyard of the yellow farmhouse and shield my eyes, turning slowly in a circle. To the south, a hill sweeps back behind the creek. To the east, another hill, encrusted with trees, climbs into the sky. You could almost reach your hand out and run your palm over it, like a closely cropped curly head. To the west, the neighbor's barn stands as the social center for gatherings of loud goats. One of the babies cries out, and for a moment I think one of my own kids is calling me.

I have a shovel in my hand. I bring it up and bury it with force into the ground. I do this four times, marking four corners of what will be my garden.

All winter I've waited for the ground to warm up so my neighbor can turn it for me. I have a tray of seeds inside under a light—for some reason, it's important that my whole garden be from seeds I started myself. Why? No one knows. I don't even know why I'm doing a garden in the first place. Some guttural urge has me out here with my hands in the dirt, my heart leaping with joy.

I've read books about gardening, and I've asked all the vegetable growers I know for advice. This time, I cannot fail. Not totally. Not like last time.

A month later, a square of brown against the green is lined with small plants. Fifteen tomato plants in four varieties, a dozen or so heirloom bell peppers. A streak of tiny shoots in the middle marks my row of sugar snap peas.

I trudge out back with a hoe. My enormous pregnant belly must look ridiculous with me hacking the ground. But the shocked pleasure has got me now—the surprising pleasure of seeing tiny baby shoots emerge from soil, neck first, unfurling as they hit the air. Every day for six weeks they've done something new, responding to light and water as fastidiously as a newborn infant adjusts to milk and cold. Now they are adjusting to the ground.

All this dirt is just liquid gold under me. I can feel the warmth when I get down on my knees to see how high the shoots have come. I have done everything I know to do this time. I spread lime over this ground to raise the PH levels after testing the soil. I spread manure from a friend's herd of goats, two-year-old manure that was nice and black. Soon I will lay down newspaper and straw to keep back the weeds. By the time the baby in my belly comes, we'll be eating dinner out of this dirt.

A month later, my baby is sleeping in a bassinet. But we've come home from the hospital to find that a heat wave killed half a dozen more tomato plants, the rest of the peppers, and all but one potato plant. It seems I didn't water them enough before we left.

The corn is doing just fine, so we borrow a special hose to slowly soak it and the dozen or so tomato plants that are left. The sugar snaps are all right—except one of the rows looks like it's being clipped from the bottom by an animal of some sort. Some of the plants on the edge are turning brown and falling. Also, I put a bunch of basil seeds straight into the ground over there—where are they? All I see is a crop of weeds coming up.

A month later, the tomatoes have been staked up and are enormous. One is taller than me. Green tomatoes everywhere—grape, roma, beefsteak. We'll have to can some. The corn is as tall as a man too, and I'm seeing the cobs getting fatter. Three of the potato plants came back from the dead and sprouted out of the dead greenery— we ate new potatoes for lunch on the fourth of July. We are swimming in basil—I've made many batches of pesto and feed it to family and friends on pizzas, on crackers, in soup, and on pasta. I'll pick more to take to my mother. My watermelon plants are starting to spread.

The sugar snap peas we got to eat for about a week, a handful a day, my daughter and I. Then the rabbits got the last of the plants. I made a trap for the rabbits with a laundry basket, a stick, and some string, but they don't seem to care for my bait at all. My husband laughed at me because he's a country boy, and he knows you can't get rabbits that way.

Every day I come out and look at my tomatoes coming in and marvel at the way the ground made them, how God made them, how he let me help. I wonder how many types of plants he's brought into being just this spring, just on our road. How many leaves did he grow this year? I saw two dozen new wildflowers come through and coat the hill, week after week, just on my road alone. What was he doing on the other roads? What is it about his personality that just spreads and overflows, grows and gives, fecundity itself?

What kind of person would I be if I could move into a farmhouse like this one on a hill like this one with a garden like this one and not marvel at it all?

The Wizard of Wheat

Norman Borlaug has been credited with saving over a billion people worldwide from starvation, and you've probably never heard his name before.

He arrived in Mexico in 1944, sent by the Rockefeller Foundation to develop disease-resistant wheat for Mexican farmers. Mexico had been hounded for years by stem rust, a quickly mutating blight that attacks wheat plants like smallpox and eats them alive. A flexible, airborne supervillain, its spores reproduce five different ways. In the 1940s, it was one of the principal reasons that Mexico was unable to feed itself.

The first year, Borlaug and two local assistants wandered around Mexican villages and snipped off about 8,000 heads of wheat. They planted 110,000 crossbred plants from those 8,600 varieties the first year. As they waited for the wheat to come up, Borlaug witnessed poverty in the local towns that he'd never seen before. Men, women, and children scratched their livings out of depleted soil with poor water access and crude farming methods.

"The solution was straightforward: bigger harvests," writes Charles Mann in his telling of the story. "More food would mean more money would mean less hunger and poverty."[2]

Borlaug spent every day of summer in 1945 walking the five miles of plants, inspecting them for stem rust and yanking out plants as soon as they showed signs of it. At the end of the year, four little rows were all they had left—four out of 110,000.

Borlaug began to believe the project was a waste of time. He could see that even if they developed a good wheat breed for the region they were in, it would be too little, too late. They couldn't address the hunger of an entire country unless they could come up with a plant that would serve any Mexican farmer in any region. Unfortunately, there was no way to do that as slowly as they were doing it. They could only raise one crop per year—right?

This was when Borlaug had the idea that would change the course of history: shuttle breeding.

He suggested to his boss in the US that he be allowed to do a crop of winter wheat in one location and then take the winners to another location in the mountains to breed it again, all within the same year. As the next few years passed, he went through stages, first breeding plants to ignore seasonal cues, then to withstand disease, then breeding them for a combination of short stalks and high yields. "Dwarf wheat" for any season or climate was the goal, and he started to see results. His plants even survived a new strain of rust that wiped out the American Wheat Belt in 1950. Over ten more years, Borlaug bred his disease-resistant, high-yielding wheat for a softer, more edible grain.

Finally, in 1960, Borlaug hosted a field day where he introduced farmers to his new superwheat. This wheat represented enormous strides in breeding technique, contributions from other scientists around the world, and 20 years of Borlaug's own life. So it came as some surprise to him when instead of being met with active enthusiasm, he was met with...apathy.

The local farmers came to hear about it, but they were skeptical. They couldn't possibly imagine the kind of research that had resulted in this magical strain of wheat. They couldn't tell the future, either—how could they know that Borlaug's semidwarf, disease-resistant varieties would utterly change the food landscape in Mexico? They didn't know that this seed of Borlaug's was an incredible gift to them and to the entire country. They rejected the gift because they had stopped looking for good things in their yearly struggle to survive. Their eyes were on the ground.[3]

A few years later, those first farmers notwithstanding, Mexico had embraced the Borlaug wheat strain. In 1963, 95 percent of Mexico's wheat crops used Borlaug's wheat. That year, the harvest was six times larger than in 1944, the year Borlaug arrived. Farmers reaped almost 2,500 pounds per acre—three times what they had gotten 20 years earlier.

Soon, Borlaug's wheat was being planted over millions of acres in India and Pakistan. Experts call this the Green Revolution—the spread of scientific victory over starvation. In Pakistan, wheat yields rose from 4.6 million tons in 1965 to 8.4 million in 1970. In India, they rose from 12.3 million tons to 20 million. And the yields continue to increase. In 2018, India harvested a record 73.5 million tons of wheat, up 11.5 percent from 1998. Since 1968, India's population has more than doubled, its wheat production has more than tripled, and its economy has multiplied nine times.

Norman Borlaug, the man who spent 20 years of his life meticulously breeding that first high-yield strain of wheat, may have saved as many as a billion human lives. He later received the Nobel Peace Prize, the Presidential Medal of Freedom, and the Congressional Gold Medal. Borlaug and other researchers like him are part of the reason why the percentage of undernourished people worldwide has dropped from 28 percent in 1970 to 11 percent in 2015,[4] even while the world population has more than doubled. They are part of the reason we have such a blessed excess of food in our grocery stores here in the US.

If we develop attitudes of apathy in the face of all this plenty, really, who can blame us? Like the farmers who encountered Borlaug's wheat in 1960, we just don't always know how to partake of good gifts when they come. They were ambivalent due to scientific misunderstanding and long years of hardship. When we are ambivalent, we don't have the same excuses. Generations of plenty have left us with another kind of ambivalence. Our apathy is perhaps not due to lack, but to plenty.

Food Apathy in a World of Plenty

The points that I underscored in previous chapters—about no ingredient being sinful, about our freedom in Christ to pursue whichever culinary course seems best to us—may have raised a host of questions in your mind. Is there a limit? You can't say it's wrong to eat gluten or dairy, but would it be wrong for a person to eat five fast-food meals a day? If we're going to make calls about what is an abuse of the body and what is just a matter of taste and opinion, are there any lines at all that we can draw?

Well, we drew lines about gluttony two chapters back. There, we called it "sin" in no uncertain terms to return again and again for the same pleasure beyond satiation and true enjoyment. In this chapter, I want to draw another line that requires careful personal application and discernment. This line has to do with whether we are culpable for continuously ignoring—refusing even to be curious about—the good things God has laid out within reach.

When we wonder aloud about whether it's a sin for somebody to eat nothing but McDonald's for the rest of their lives, we should at least ask what kind of sin might be on the table for consideration. Are we talking about a sin of abuse? The body as a temple and all that? Are we talking about the sin of gluttony? Or is it possible that we could also explore this question under another, less-talked-of sin? What about the sin of apathy?

G.K. Chesterton famously said that the world will never starve for want of wonders, but for want of wonder.[5] Is it possible for us—particularly we Christians, who supposedly see the created world as a product of God's pen and paintbrush—is it possible for any of us to reach a point where we are sinning in our refusal to take note of it?

A man who walks past his first glimpse of the Grand Canyon without stopping to look must have something wrong going on in his heart or head. But what about the man who lives near the Grand Canyon and passes it on his way to work? He can't be amazed every time. Still, for him to reach a point when it never takes his breath away, surely this would be a sign that his senses had been deadened.

It's right to enjoy the enjoyable. It's right to praise the praiseworthy. We should be capable of noticing things that are worthy of notice. And that includes the creek that follows me down my road when I'm driving anywhere from my rural home, the unexpected spectacle of a wasp that somebody caught under a wine glass at a party I was at recently, and the experience of whipped cream and strawberry jam on top of a perfectly turned out, barely sweetened scone.

We shouldn't be people who are dead to these pleasures. Why? Because God made them. Also, because he richly provides them to enjoy (1 Timothy 6:17). Also, because the kind of person who doesn't care when they encounter something beautiful or enjoyable is *the kind of person who doesn't care when they encounter God.*

I don't mean at all to imply that the virtue of noticing and enjoying is a virtue that leads us directly to God. As far as character traits go, it's one of the ones that is an easy sell. Anyone, whether they love God or not, can resolve to develop their eye for detail and their taste for the tasty. It isn't even one of those secular virtues that sounds *hard*—like unselfishness, for instance, or becoming organized.

So no, learning to appreciate good food isn't necessarily going to get us closer to God. But can they be related at all? What is the relationship between the ability to see and enjoy matter, and the ability to see and enjoy God? Can one awaken the other?

I would say that while tasting well doesn't necessarily lead us into worshiping God, worshiping God necessarily leads us to taste well. The muscles of tasting and seeing get used in the muscles of worship. Becoming less apathetic about the physical things God gives us is a natural by-product of becoming less apathetic about God himself.

"The creation of food, tongues, and the human digestive system is the product of infinite wisdom knitting the world together in a harmonious whole," writes Joe Rigney. "The symphony of glory that sounds from the triune being contains notes of corn salsa and Sour Patch Kids, of sweet tea and rye bread...The variety of tastes creates categories and gives us edible images of divine things."[6]

A lover of God becomes slowly more awake to good, beautiful, and enjoyable things, not less so. Lovers of God can get more out of less. They can give thanks over pleasures so simple and ordinary that others might overlook them. Their enjoyment is not the clutching enjoyment of a glutton or a miser; it's the enjoyment of a child sitting in front of something his father made for him especially. It's freely felt, free in the knowledge that because of the Father we have, there's more where this came from. We can give thanks for this leaf and enjoy it without stress. There are thousands more. This doesn't lead us to take the leaf in our hands for granted; it drives us to study the leaf and find out what our Father thought was so worthwhile that he made billions of them.

Perhaps this virtue is easier to recognize when it's missing. We know it instinctively: The apathetic person is missing something. The apathetic person can't be a worshiper. And a person who's apathetic about God's creation has surely missed some aspect of what it means to love God himself.

Richly All Things to Enjoy

Problems with apathy always arise in the midst of plenty. The starving man has no problem noticing his full plate. But in a time and place where most of us have more than we need (this applies to almost every category of living, from entertainment to food to space), apathy hounds us. How can we really care about a nice meal when we're sure to have another one tomorrow morning?

When Paul addresses rich people in his letter to Timothy, he's talking to us. We are the rich people, and we're still trying to figure out what to do with our abundance:

> As for the rich in this present age, charge them not to be haughty, nor to set their hopes on the uncertainty of riches, but on God, who richly provides us with everything to enjoy. They are to do good, to be rich in good works, to be generous and ready to share, thus storing up treasure for themselves as a good foundation for the future, so that they may take hold of that which is truly life (1 Timothy 6:17-19).

Notice that Paul doesn't say, "Charge them not to be haughty, nor to set their hopes on the uncertainty of riches, but on God, *who will make sure they don't have material experiences that distract from his goodness.*" Neither does he say, "They are to do good, be rich in good works, *and avoid material pleasure when possible.*"

Rather, he warns us not to set our hopes on the uncertainty of riches or on the things that riches provide (conveniences, comforts, sensory experiences). And then he says to be rich in good works and to set our hope on God, "who richly provides us with everything to enjoy."

Is this something along the logical line of "set your sights on heaven, and you get earth thrown in; set your sights on earth, and you get neither"? Not quite, I don't think. The promises of God are to attract us for their own sake; we are to long for God because he intends us to discover more and more fully over time that he himself is the overflowing possession we seek. I think it contradicts the logic of this passage to argue, "Set your sights on God, and guess what? He'll give you good stuff if you do."

But Paul does mention, very deliberately, and at an odd moment, the things that God gives us to enjoy. He mentions them in the same breath with warning us not to set our hope on them. So why does he mention them at all? Why remind us—at the moment of telling us to store up riches in heaven by loosening our grasp on earthly riches—why remind us that God is a God who happens to enjoy excessive displays of blessing? *And that he intends for us to enjoy the things when he gives them?*

I believe Paul's wording is deliberate. He wants us (even us rich people) to have the full picture of the kind of God we serve. We are commanded to let go of material things and set our sights on God, but we should always keep in our minds a picture of God as an openhanded God. He is a God of limits and of freedoms, a God of "no" and "yes," a God of waiting and a God of fulfilling. But if we want to know what the final note of God's character will be, it must always contain a predominate note of prosperity and showered blessing. Because the story that he's telling will end *there*. It won't end with the no, but with the yes. It won't end with the wait, but with the fulfillment. It won't end with the pain of limits, but with the glory of freedoms within limits that feel natural. In the end, he plans to wine and dine us on himself. He plans to bless the socks off of his people.

So even when we are disciplining our hearts not to love things with inordinate love, we must constantly remember that the God we're supposed to turn our hearts to is, come to find out, the same God "who richly provides us with everything to enjoy."

The Beekeeper

My father-in-law is a beekeeper. One day this summer, we drove our van out to the hives and pulled the children into the front seat so they could see the bees. Rue Alan came out, clad all in white, face barely visible under the veiled hood, gloved and booted like some woodsy moon man. He held a wooden frame in his hands and brought it straight over to the driver side window. It was teeming with bees.

In perfect symmetry, hexagonal compartments covered the frame's two sides. He showed us which ones held sleeping eggs, which ones were filled with liquid honey. As he pointed and shouted identifiers through the glass, the bees never stopped moving, crawling, flying, buzzing. A mass of gold, building and guarding a mass of gold.

I later followed Rue Alan inside to see the purification process. Stacks of boxes and frames sat in one corner of the outbuilding. He described the process by which a queen is made, when nurse bees coddle and feed one egg with that magic called royal jelly. When she starts laying, she can produce 2,000 eggs a day. Her production slows after a year or so, and by instinct, the workers decide to raise a new queen. Sometimes, if a hive grows too big, the workers become church planters—they split down the middle, and half the workers head out to produce a new queen and start a new colony.

Rue Alan says he's often seen the dance that bees do, when they are communicating pollen sources to each other. They fly side to side, up and down, and vary the size of their dances, in order to tell each other where to go and what kind of pollen can be found in that location.

He's also witnessed them follow their queen in marching formation. When he finds a natural hive and decides to move it into his wooden boxes, he must suit up and cut the hanging hive from the tree. And from above, he says, there's no sight like it—the queen drops down in the hive, and the others swarm in an orderly fashion after her. They know their duty, and their duty is to stay with their queen.

I picked up a frame and peered into it. The frames were stored in the hive in an upright position. Each hexagon of paper-thin wax had been built by the worker bees at a slight angle, rather than being straight to the side. Why? Because it's a tiny cup to hold honey, of course. It's built at an angle so the honey won't fall out.

Rue Alan explained the process to me:

> Each of these frames gets put into an expensive stainless-steel machine shaped like an enormous drum. This machine spins the frames to strip honey and honeycomb together out of the frames. Then this messy mixture goes into another machine, which strains out the honeycomb and warms the honey, allowing it to flow through pipes into another area, which strains it, and then strains it one last time before it flows into a 100-gallon tank. The tank has a lid and a spigot, and the men use this spigot to fill bottles—mostly quarts but some gallons. They sell it cheap for pure local honey, and there's always a waiting list.

I peeked into the vat, and 80 gallons of liquid glory shone up at me. I walked over and stared at the mass of sticky honeycomb crumbles in another machine—there must have been hundreds of pounds of it in one vat alone, waiting to be bottled separately or stripped to make beeswax candles—and the absolute value of it floored me. *It's totally inimitable,* I thought. *Only bees can do this.*

Only beekeepers have access to it. Each bee only makes 1/12 of a teaspoon of honey in their lifetime. And yet, look what can be done by all of them in nonstop motion.

I had been using this honey up, gratefully pouring it on oatmeal for my girls and baking it into bread for guests, and it just kept on coming. At the end of the spring and fall robbing seasons (when beekeepers "rob" the bees of their honey, leaving enough for the hive to live off of), Rue Alan would always set a box on our counter with four or five shining bottles inside, in varying seasonal shades of amber.

Like everyone who gets free gifts and doesn't know anything about what they cost, I had no idea of the process that brought this sweet, sticky stuff to my door. I just ate it. So learning more about the process made the gift that much sweeter.

And do you think I'll ever be able to buy honey in a store again without my heart sinking a little? Can you imagine if I had bottles of this stuff in my pantry and went to Walmart for corn syrup and poured it all over my pancakes? Once you understand the value of something good, it changes the way you consume that thing. You taste it more fully, and you are better able to love it for what it is—and for the person who brought it to you.

Food can be like this, and maybe it should be like this whenever possible. Acquiring food has been a process for a long time, and just because we have ways of shortcutting the process now doesn't mean the shortcut should always be taken. It certainly doesn't mean that the shortcut will always result in the same end product.

Seeing the value of food doesn't mean we can't look at food as fuel sometimes and be grateful that peanut butter and jelly sandwiches are an easy option. But surely, as we grow in our awareness of God, we should be willing to also grow in our awareness of what he's given and how he's seen fit to give it. Peanut butter and jelly all day every day would be a sad failure to recognize what has become available to us, through a strange process of economic and farming breakthroughs. God has made much more available to us than peanut butter and jelly—especially if we're willing to get curious and learn some new skills. And he didn't make bees and give them an insane work ethic so that we could yawn and reach for the Mrs. Butterworth's.

Experiments in Noticing and Enjoying

Robert Capon put a parable in *The Supper of the Lamb* that illustrates the problem of a person who's incapable of appreciating food. In the parable, a widow and a single man are both invited to a supper party. The host intends to set them up. But his friends tell him he's crazy; these two people couldn't be more different. The widow starts talking about how much she wishes there were more kinds of meat; she gets bored cooking only beef, pork, chicken, and lamb. Then the single man starts talking about how, if he were in charge of creation, he would make it so that no one had to bother with all this "uneconomical riot of flora and fauna." He would prefer just one animal and one type of vegetation to keep the carbon cycle going. The two people are entranced with each other and leave the party engrossed in conversation.

The host smiles and explains that what they had in common was total lack of the playful spirit. Both of them were unable to be thankful for the vast variety of ingredients available to them: she because she couldn't see their potential, and he because he didn't want variety in the first place. They'd soon start living off of nutritional meal supplements, Capon says, and bless people by not burdening dinner parties with their tedious conversation.[7]

The playful spirit is something that Capon values highly, perhaps more highly than he should. But we have to admit that without some measure of this sense of fun, the kitchen becomes a burden-some place indeed. Especially for the wife and mother who has to feed people three times a day, seven days a week. For many women, food is a job, and not one that they chose voluntarily. More on that in another chapter.

If abundance makes it difficult to practice seeing and enjoying, grunt work makes it difficult as well. You can't delight in the subtle play of jelly on peanut butter—not every week. You can't keep up a sense of enthralled wonder in the texture of chili on cornbread—not if you're going to stay sane. The material thing is that your fam-ily needs to eat something, and they need it tonight. Is there time for "the playful spirit"? Is there time to notice the flavors of God's cre-ation when other members of his creation—namely, your husband and kids—are in a very present need of some spaghetti?

Not every meal can transport us to a place of gratitude and grace. But what I'm advocating for here is practice. More and more, we should be eating food that allows us to thank God heartily before, during, and after eating it. This has to do with a heart attitude and a habit of gratitude for things besides food. But it also has to do with what we're eating—to a certain extent.

C.S. Lewis wrote in *An Experiment in Criticism* that the defi-nition of a good book was a book that could be read *in the right way*.[8] He meant that only a good book can be read thoughtfully and repeatedly. I think the same idea could be helpfully applied to food. Good food is food that can be eaten the right way.

I can't imagine sitting down and really mulling over a Twinkie (perhaps someone could), but I can imagine sitting down to a French pastry made with real butter and giving my full attention to it, washing it down with coffee and gratitude. I have never had a good experience with ice cream that comes in a large plastic tub with a handle (perhaps someone has). But I have had several memorable experiences with a single or double scoop of cherry-chocolate ice cream made out of real cream—experiences that left me feeling like I'd done a good thing (rather than feeling like I'd just ingested hydrogenated dairy substitute and that it was lingering in a film on my tongue).

The nutritional profile of these foods isn't necessarily the main thing that divides them in the examples I just mentioned. You could use real butter and still make a sorry pastry with it. But in each case, I cannot imagine eating the first food the way food ought to be eaten—with thanksgiving and relish. And I can imagine eating the second that way.

So perhaps the first step in addressing food apathy is to practice the same impulses we are strengthening in fighting gluttony: the impulse that can distinguish between food that is taken with thanksgiving and food that is taken in mindless habit.

It's also true that apathy is on the opposite end from the sin we talked about in the last chapter—snobbery. You can start caring about your ingredients so much and noticing them so thoroughly that you're incapable of graciously consuming fast food when it's being served. But on the other hand, you can become a person who isn't even curious what there is to eat besides fast food. Or perhaps can't taste the difference between a home-cooked meal and a frozen dinner.

The point is that in this area, like in the area of gluttony, a stronger sense of taste will help us. And that can be developed through the practice of paying attention.

Another Kind of Apathy

So far, I've avoided addressing some of the ethical questions that arise as we stock our pantries and refrigerators. I made a brief reference to them at the end of the first chapter: *What about the environment—are we responsible if the food we consume is produced in ways that damage resources? What about animal welfare—are we responsible if the animals we consume were mistreated? What about fair-trade practices—what if the food we eat is only on our table because somebody was paid too little for their product?*

I want to be very careful here, because the entire thrust of this book is to relieve obligation to man-made rules around food and encourage freedom in the Holy Spirit. So I'm not going to give you new laws here, such as "Don't eat GMO wheat," "Don't eat industrial beef," "Don't drink coffee unless it's fair trade." These are enormous topics with data that constantly changes year by year. So instead of addressing details and specific practices, I'll offer a few observations that guide my decision-making around these questions:

1. You are responsible for what you know, but you can't know everything.

In general, our tendency today is to take too much responsibility for things that are outside our control (i.e., the precise sourcing of every product that enters our homes), and too little responsibility for things that we're very much responsible for (i.e., our hearts, our tongues, etc.). So, if you release some of that low-grade guilt you might carry over all the stuff you should be doing that you can't do, the stuff you should be reading about that you can't read about, it may free you up to take responsibility for what you know (i.e., your duty to love and serve your neighbor and do it joyfully).

2. We are stewards of creation.

The fact is, humans are in charge around here, and we are responsible for how we take care of our animals and our land. The land and the animals are not gods unto themselves, to be served—they are in fact made for us, not the other way around. But we know we were given a mandate to take good care of our things. God has given humanity dominion over the works of his hands, says the psalmist; he has "put all things under his feet, all sheep and oxen, and also the beasts of the field, the birds of the heavens, and the fish of the sea, whatever passes along the paths of the seas" (Psalm 8:6-8).

3. Good stewards are blessed, and bad stewards experience consequences.

The questions of whether animals should be raised in CAFOs (concentrated animal feeding operations) and whether mass production of corn and soy is a good idea depend on a great many factors, and there are lots of expert opinions, many of which conflict. But we can safely assume that where humankind is careless about the things God put under our stewardship, we can expect consequences. If it's a bad idea to pump animals full of hormones and give them less than optimal time to grow, you might expect to see a negative change in the chemical makeup of their meat. If you drain soil of nutritional value by relentlessly pulling food from it without husbanding it back to health, you should experience poor (or at least, mixed) results.

4. There are constantly multiplying factors for the steward to consider.

But it's also helpful to remember why these questions are so hard to answer. Other principles are at work, economic principles of trade-offs. For instance, is it better for millions of people to starve, or for those same people to eat GMOs and live? Is it better for meat to be scarce and high quality, or plentiful and low quality? Is it better to get plentiful crops by killing bugs with pesticides, or for fewer people to have access to green vegetables, and for those vegetables to be pesticide free? It's helpful to keep in mind that for every voiced opinion on these matters, there is usually an equal and opposite opinion to be taken into consideration. This is why the reading can be so exhausting, and why when we make value statements, they should be nuanced and lightly held.

5. Where knowledge makes us responsible, we should pay people what they're worth.

Ephesians 4:28 reads, "Let the thief no longer steal, but rather let him labor, doing honest work with his own hands, so that he may have something to share with anyone in need." From this verse, we can draw helpful guidelines for fair-trade practices. If you have no idea what I'm talking about when you read the phrase "fair-trade coffee," I'm not trying to press a charge of stealing on you. But imagine you've been catching an article here and a news report there, and somehow you hear that the coffee you've been buying by the truckload is sourced in a village where all the coffee farmers are near starvation because prices have been driven so low. And around the same time, you hear that a man in your church started a coffee business designed to source coffee at fair prices from specific regions that he has personally visited. Now imagine his coffee is more expensive (of course it is). You probably ought to look into it. This feels like a similar situation to the one addressed by Paul in 1 Corinthians 10:27-29, when he advises readers to eat freely of food that was used in idol worship, but if someone brings new information to you, pay attention, and perhaps abstain.

There's also a great deal of difference between you swindling your local farmer's market farmer by lying about how many pounds of tomatoes you put in your trunk and buying tomatoes at Walmart without knowing which farm they came from. The bottom line for these questions of ethical responsibility is one of weight. Should you become a person who preaches these values without acknowledging how complicated they are? Should you start acting like ecological questions are central to the gospel? Absolutely not. But neither should you pretend that you don't vote with your dollar, that your opinion is totally private and has no moral ramifications. You aren't a dietary agnostic, remember. You are a steward.

You don't have to take on the weight of the world. Perhaps small adjustments are exactly what is needed. Perhaps you could eat less beef and enjoy better beef when you do. Perhaps you could enjoy some of the bounty offered by your local farms, making it a fun challenge to incorporate what you find there. Don't sit around feeling guilty for something you don't understand. Make the best decisions you can, based on your knowledge, and let go of the rest.

"The earth is the LORD's, and the fullness thereof" (Psalm 24:1).

How to Eat a Pomegranate

Pomegranates are my favorite fruit. They have been my favorite since the year I turned 13.

Formerly, my favorite fruit was mango. Unfortunately for me, the year I turned 13 was the year my father bought an entire case of mangos because they were on deep sale, which I proceeded to devour to the tune of four or five a day (moderation for me, always moderation). Apparently, it's possible to develop an allergy to something by eating far too much of it. A few days in, I developed a bizarre reaction on the lower half of my face—a kind of rash that stayed put and eventually turned dry and flaky and numb before finally disappearing. I laid off on the mango for a while, but months later, when I ate just one, the rash returned around my lips.

My favorite fruit was ruined for me forever. So, I decided that my second favorite fruit, pomegranate, would have to be moved up to first place. And this was more than 15 years ago, well before the superfood pome-craze of the early 2010s. It was a fruit deserving of affection long before the pomegranate shampoo people got to it.

If you haven't spent any personal time with a pomegranate, it's time for you to do so. Pick one up in your hands at the grocery store. It's a richer red than most apples you meet, and larger. It looks from a distance to be perfectly round, but on closer inspection, it's imperfectly round; it has a series of plateaus that combine to make a round whole. Your mind wants to register it as slightly shriveled because of that imperfect shape, but pick it up. It has the shiny, firm, waxy skin to prove that it's bursting with newness.

On top of the pomegranate (or actually the bottom, according to the direction it hangs on the fruit tree), there is a crown-like structure. It looks like an extreme outie belly button that stretched until it burst. Take this pomegranate home.

Take it to your kitchen table and sit down with it. You're going to be here for a while, so get nice and comfortable. Set a nice, wide plate down as a workspace, and next to it a bowl that is beautiful enough to hold the royal fruit.

Get yourself a good scoring knife. Open the proceedings by putting one score around the exterior of the fruit. You may also hold the fruit with its belly button away from you and view it from above. You'll notice that those misshapen plateaus are actually quite regulated; there are six of them. Instead of one score all the way around, you could make six scores down the sides of the pomegranate, on the ridges between these six plateaus, as if you were scoring the earth into sections that had pointy tips at the North Pole and the South.

Your score must not be more than a few millimeters deep—maybe as much as a centimeter. You're just trying to get through the waxy skin and perhaps a bit of the pulpy layer of "fat" just underneath it.

After the score, use your fingers at the belly button crown to pry the fruit apart. It should come willingly. It is already given to separation within, though the system of pulpy chambers and the tough rind give it a stability and protection not to be rivaled by any custom Styrofoam packing system.

When you open it, your breath may catch in your throat for a moment. Perfect sheets, or hills, or mounds of pomegranate seeds lie packed within this system. Their color is the first thing that shocks you. You can see why the poet who wrote the Song of Solomon reached for these exquisite "cheeks" of untapped potential when he was describing his mate ("Your cheeks are like halves of a pomegranate behind your veil..." [Song of Solomon 4:3]).

Peel away the papery layer over the top of them, and begin to pop them—gently, gently, with the pads of your thumbs—out of their pulp-Styrofoam backing. Individually, you'll find that they look very much like brilliantly red kernels of corn. Bite one in half, and you'll find that it is like a packet of juice, with a tiny seed in the center that delivers a crunch. Continue your work until the bowl is full. It will be not much more than a cup of seeds to one pomegranate. Each seed could ruin your shirt. If you have done your job properly, the bowl will be mainly dry, and the seeds will still feel like fresh corn kernels before they've been removed from the cob, not slippery to the touch in their own juice.

Take a spoon and dip it into the mound of seeds (actually, these are "arils"—individual juice containers for the real seed). Take a full bite of them. Take your time in crushing the arils in one mouthful. This is, in my opinion, the best way to eat a pomegranate, although many like to let it last by fingering and nibbling just a few arils at a time. They are also delightful in salads and combined with chocolate. But this here is my vote—the slow eating with a spoon out of a bowl that deserves to hold them.

Now, if this is your delight in the pomegranate, imagine God's delight in it. He who designed the custom Styrofoam packing system to contain his pristine arils of scarlet juice. He who knows the chamber design in each of these globes before they are scored and cracked open.[9] Worship-worthy creative glory can be found, you see, not only on the macro level. It is just as astounding in micro form.

FOOD FOR THOUGHT

Discuss

- Are you more like the lady in the parable who thought there wasn't enough variety in creation to keep from being bored, or the man who thought it would be better if there was only one type of animal and one type of vegetation to live off of?

- Why do you think God didn't just make our bodies to need tasteless nutrition packets, delivered intravenously or via the sun? What on earth could be the meaning of all this variety?

- Of the ethical questions discussed in this chapter, which do you find the most overwhelming? Do you feel after reading that you might be responsible to learn more or to make any adjustments based on what you know?

Practice

- Plant a garden. Grow something in a planter or in your own backyard. Tomatoes and basil are a great place to start. They grow well in most places and can both contribute to a summer of Italian cooking.

- Take a field trip to a local food source—where you can watch a process or participate. Visit a pick-your-own berry farm or apple orchard, visit a farm where you can see what it looks like to grow a variety of crops, look up your local beekeeper's association, or watch a friend make jam. You develop your appreciation for God's provided bounty when you see the process.

- Dissect a pomegranate.

Read

- Read *The Things of Earth* by Joe Rigney for a discussion of material things and why it's okay to enjoy them in light of eternity.

PART 2

FEASTING *for* ETERNITY

CHAPTER 5

Hospitality

LOVE IN THE POT

"Go therefore to the main roads and invite to the wedding feast as many as you find." And those servants went out into the roads and gathered all whom they found, both bad and good. So the wedding hall was filled with guests.

—MATTHEW 22:9-10

From Memory: 2018

I'm stirring with a metal spoon, reaching into an enormous pot that contains nothing but oil and flour. One cup of each, in the bottom of the pot, slowly stirring between bouts of chopping vegetables. The veggies are three: onions, green peppers, and celery. They have been called the holy trinity of Cajun cooking.

In the pot, the mixture grows warm colored, moving from muddy white to raw sienna to burnt sienna to burnt umber. The burnt umber gives way to what my father helpfully describes as milk chocolate. This is to be distinguished from dark chocolate. It's a helpful distinction because you must absolutely wait for the moment milk gives way to dark. You must not stop too soon. Also, you can never leave the pot during this time, or you'll end up with a black coat of ruinous film on the bottom and have to start over.

The moment the roux is the color of dark chocolate, I run over to get the enormous holy trinity bowl of vegetables, and I throw it in and coat those vegetables all over with the dark chocolate. And they miraculously stop the process of darkening, faster than it could ever be stopped if I just pulled the pot off the heat. Not only that, but the oil in the roux begins to cook them instantly. They sauté evenly, even though there is what feels like a third of a pot of them. They begin to release their juices.

With the moment of crisis passed, I'm no longer chained to the stove top. I move to where a whole chicken is lying on a blue plate. It has been boiled and cooled; the stock is waiting to be strained directly into the pot.

I pull a breast off, remove its skin. I shred the meat. I pick the entire chicken clean. My carnivorous three-year-old finds out and comes up to the counter to steal a mouthful of dark meat.

I slice a good Cajun-style smoked sausage and put it in a pan to brown. All of this will go into the enormous pot together and simmer for an hour or two. It will be best refrigerated or frozen for later. Because gumbo is always best the second day.

Tomorrow, I'll cook an enormous pot of rice, and the people will come for gumbo night. Every Friday night, I try to feed three families including ours. I try to bring people from the church together with people outside the church. I try to bring big families full of children together with older couples who have passed their childbearing years. I try to bring singles together with marrieds.

The gumbo is not a trick, but it is a sort of bargain. I feed them to get them into the house, and then keep them there with conversation. Everyone has to huddle in the same room because our house is small—the dining table seats six, so overflow folks sit on couches and chairs nearby. Bowls are balanced on knees with hunks of bread nearby.

The gumbo is the open door, but the gumbo is not the point.

Feeding as the Prelude to Gospel Fellowship

It's amazing how much people love to be fed. Not even to be fed fancy food—just food they didn't have to think about, buy, or cook themselves.

When my friend makes me a salad for lunch because I happen to be at her house and hungry, I feel loved. I crow with delight when she asks me if I want ice cream with the Arnold Palmer cake she made. The salad could be identical to one I make at home (although it never is, with salads; that's what's so great about someone making a salad for you), but it would taste better. This is how I know someone cares—they sliced tomatoes for me.

And if you start to get this into your mind—people feel love in the food you make—you'll begin to use the food as a means of showing love. You'll be cooking and serving strategically, with a gospel-driven love that sees food as a means to an end. People are not a means to an end. Not even the end of making converts or building influence. But food can be a means to love people. Food can purchase an audience to talk about the things that matter to both of you.

On Tuesdays this summer, I've been bringing the teen girls in the church to my house to go through a study of Hebrews. They were eager and ready to do something of this kind, and their sweet requests moved me to put some other summer plans aside and make it happen.

They come in the afternoon, and if everyone makes it, we have 12 there. So, of course, as part of the teatime ritual, I make a blueberry coffeecake for them. It is a delight to my soul to lay tea and cake out for these girls every Tuesday. On the one hand, it's a delight that these are still girls, and they're not squeamish about eating a bit of sugar in the afternoon—the cake is usually eaten to the last crumb. Also, they are all serious tea drinkers, come to find out. We sometimes polish off three pots. Last week I wasn't able to bake anything and was just getting home from grocery shopping when they arrived, so they helped me unpack the groceries, and then we shared a bar of chocolate over Hebrews chapter 10.

This kind of unfussiness, and seeing teen girls politely tear into a blueberry coffeecake, gives me a wonderful sense of God's pleasure. Because once we sit down with our teacups, we open the Word and attempt to understand and apply one of the most rich and difficult books in the Bible. They are feeding with me on the Word, and what kind of teen girls are willing to spend their summers pushing through these passages? The teatime is not what keeps them coming—they asked for a study before teatime was imagined—but it's a perfect accompaniment to the hard work that we are doing.

And if I managed to sit around with these girls for days and weeks over tea without study, without talking about the things that matter most to our souls, I would have wasted a good coffee cake. It would be entirely possible to have tea without deriving any spiritual benefit at all. But when we use hospitality as an aid and a vehicle for intimacy and truth and worship, we are using it as it was intended to be used, and as I think it will be used in the new heavens and new earth.

In Rebekah Merkle's words, we are "enfleshing" the gospel with these little homey rituals:

> It's not that men are supposed to be involved in teaching theology and women aren't—it's that men are to teach it one way and women are to teach it another. If men are the words, women are the music. If men are the skeletons, women are the flesh. If men are the radio waves, women are the amplifiers...[1]

> Our job as women—and it's a phenomenal responsibility—is to enflesh the weighty truths of our faith. If our role is to make truth taste, to make holiness beautiful,

then what does that look like in the details? As a random example of this, take Christmas. Christmas is, of course, when God did, ultimately, what we women can only shadow. The ultimate enfleshing...The men can talk about the Incarnation, church fathers can write important treatises about it, pastors can preach about it, theologians can parse and define it...but we women are the ones who make it taste like something. We make it smell good.[2]

...And for my next trick, I will take Athanasius' *De Incarnatione* and I will say it with cookies and wrapping paper and cinnamon and marshmallows and colored lights and tablecloths and shopping trips and frantically-last-minute-late-night-Amazon-orders and ham—and I will do it in such a way that my four-year-old will really get it, and it will send roots deep down into his soul where it will anchor his loves and his loyalties and shape his allegiances well into his nineties.[3]

Our work in setting up a place where teatimes and gumbo nights can happen is our way of making the truth into something you can experience viscerally. You can taste joy, touch joy, smell joy—and the work of the woman who cares about both truth and taste is capable of working both of the crucial elements of Christian hospitality.

In *The Gospel Comes with a House Key*, Rosaria Butterfield describes her own breakneck schedule of hospitality and preparation for hospitality, represented by lists of tasks. Then she says:

My lists are not set in stone; they are set in grace, organized around people and their needs and their special pain and deep wounds and unbearable secrets. Some of my lists look like common grocery lists, but that is only if you see the surface of things. Committing your life to good neighboring is both art and science...

The upshot of all these lists is when, after dinner, the
Bible and the Psalters open and Kent teaches, and we—a
shabby, makeshift "we" of people, neighbors and God's
family all tossed together in a heap—listen, question,
weep, sing, laugh, receive, and pray...all these lists lead
to this moment, when strangers are rendered brothers
and sisters in Christ, heads bowed; when the Holy Spirit
drives, Jesus speaks, and we receive.[4]

But I'd Rather Just Cook

I have a friend who is shy, and the most incredible event plan-
ner you'd ever meet. When a dinner, luncheon, or shower is being
planned by the church, it's likely that she is the one running things
behind the scenes. She knows what it takes to get the place deco-
rated, get the right dishes in and out in one piece. She can make
dozens of finger sandwiches and have them ready at the same time
as the gluten-free crackers and cheese, the blueberry and cucumber
water, the banana Portuguese custard tarts.

But my friend is shy. She hides her shyness behind a brisk busy-
ness, but it often defines her social experiences. Because of this, my
friend knows that it would be easy for her to tend to the details and
then step back and pretend that her work was done when the real,
live people arrived. They would enjoy the fruit of her hands. But, in
the end, she could be guilty of addressing their bodies and ignoring
their souls.

A hostess who loves her guests is still present when the food preparation is done and the eating has begun. She was loving her guests
to prepare all those custard tarts. But when the custard tarts are in
their tray, she must still be in the mode of loving, even when more
interpersonal kinds of love are especially taxing for her.

Jen Wilkin helpfully points out distinctions between hospitality and what she calls "entertaining."

> Entertaining involves setting the perfect tablescape after an exhaustive search on Pinterest. It chooses a menu that will impress, and then frets its way through each stage of preparation. It requires every throw pillow to be in place, every cobweb to be eradicated, every child to be neat and orderly. It plans extra time to don the perfect outfit before the first guest touches the doorbell on the seasonally decorated doorstep. And should any element of the plan fall short, entertaining perceives the entire evening to have been tainted. Entertaining focuses attention on self.
>
> Hospitality involves setting a table that makes everyone feel comfortable. It chooses a menu that allows face time with guests instead of being chained to the stovetop. It picks up the house to make things pleasant but doesn't feel the need to conceal evidences of everyday life. It sometimes sits down to dinner with flour in its hair. It allows the gathering to be shaped by the quality of the conversation rather than the cuisine. Hospitality shows interest in the thoughts, feelings, pursuits, and preferences of its guests. It is good at asking questions and listening intently to answers. Hospitality focuses attention on others.[5]

Our hospitality has to be about serving people and worshiping God. A wise woman knows that people have both bodies and souls, and that she can serve both of those with the warmth of femininity God gave her. Loving people through hospitality means drawing them into intimacy with conversation. We must become practiced not just in getting the bread out on time, but in reflexively referencing the God who gives bread in abundance. Our talk must be salted (and so, absolutely, should our soup). This is what makes for the kind of hospitality that gives life—rather than leaching it out, one perfectly browned crème brûlée and barren, worldly conversation at a time.

Ferial and Festal Eating

Father Capon puts forth a distinction in his exuberant book *The Supper of the Lamb* that will be helpful for our thinking about hospitality. He says that instead of diet food and fattening food, we should have two categories of eating that we alternate between: ferial and festal.

Ferial eating is everyday eating. It is what you serve your family on weekdays, and guests when they are especially close friends. You can invite the Smiths over and feed them the same bean-and-cheese quesadillas that you always feed the family on Thursday night.

Festal eating is the special occasion, the feast. It is your expensive ingredients, your meal that requires an RSVP because you have to know exactly how many of the little bacon-wrapped asparagus packets to make. It is the Christmas, the Thanksgiving, the dinner party. It is once in a while, and if you try to eat it more often than once in a while, you find that it loses its savor. "For everything there is a season," says the Preacher. "A time to weep, and a time to laugh; a time to mourn, and a time to dance...a time to embrace, and a time to refrain from embracing" (Ecclesiastes 3:1,4-5). A time to eat steak, and time to eat beans.

Capon describes the two cuisines: "To the extraordinary or festal cuisine are relegated all roasts, joints, chops and steaks, and, in general, any meats that are cooked in large pieces and carved at the table. To the ferial cuisine belong all the rest—the dishes which take a little, cut it up small, and make it go a long way."[6] Accompanying this advice, as the backbone of his book, Capon offers his recipe for "Lamb for Eight Persons Four Times," which is his direction for cooking one leg of lamb so that it feeds literally eight people on four separate occasions. This involves stew made with good wine, sauce made with good fat, and lots of potatoes or pasta to carry the whole thing along.

I bring this up in a conversation about hospitality because it strikes me that we need a distinction like this to practice hospitality well and not kill ourselves in the process. I don't mean that ferial eating should be lazy and cheerless—if anything, the budget-stretcher cuisines are some of the most delicious and require as much skill as any other. Fresh pasta? Ferial cuisine. Gumbo? Ferial. Garlic mashed potatoes? Ferial, unless accompanied by a whole lamb chop. Capon comments:

> The poor man may envy the rich their houses, their lands, and their cars; but given a good wife, he rarely envies them their table. The rich man dines festally, but unless he is an exceptional lover of being—unless he has the soul of a poet and a saint—his feasts are too often only single: They delight the palate, but not the intellect. They are greeted with a deluxe but mindless attention: "What was it, dear, sirloin or porterhouse?" Every dish in the ferial cuisine, however, provides a double or treble delight: Not only is the body nourished and the palate pleased, the mind is intrigued by the triumph of ingenuity over scarcity—by the making of slight materials into a considerable matter. A man can do worse than be poor.[7]

The ferial cuisines that Capon is talking about here just involve feeding numbers of people out of one pot rather than carving everybody a ten-ounce portion of meat, complete with three sides and a dinner roll. One-pot cooking is the stuff that life is made of. And, usually, it's a pot full of carbs. Beans, rice, grain, and potatoes have kept people alive from the Edenic exile until now. If we learn to do this cuisine well, we'll be able to feed our families and our friends without fuss for years to come. But if we get stuck in a land of place cards and matching wine glasses, we'll never have anybody over.

Everyday hospitality doesn't mean sloppy cooking. But it can mean skilled use of resources to make a little go a long way, and to let the heavy lifting be done by good old standbys.

The Dinner Party

There's another reason to get good at ferial cooking that we don't have to think so hard about. In addition to helping us to be more hospitable in general, it'll free us up to plan the menu for that special dinner party we've been waiting to throw. When the time does come, nobody is more gleefully ready for a special celebration than Capon. At the end of his book, he offers his own best advice for throwing a good dinner party for eight.

> First, the dinner party is a true proclamation of the abundance of being—a rebuke to the thrifty little idolatries by which we lose sight of the lavish hand that made us. It is precisely because no one needs soup, fish, meat, salad, cheese, and dessert at one meal that we so badly need to sit down to them from time to time. It was *largesse* that made us all; we were not created to fast forever. The unnecessary is the taproot of our being and the last key to the door of delight. Enter here, therefore, as a sovereign remedy for the narrowness of our minds and the stinginess of our souls, the formal dinner for six, eight or ten chosen guests, the true *convivium*—the long Session that brings us nearly home.[8]

Capon's view of the dinner party as an expression of God's abundance gave me a new perspective. We are created for a future of solemn, kingly enjoyment of "the lavish hand that made us." Surely, even for pilgrims and sojourners, there is room here on earth for occasions that hearken forward to that future. So, in reading Capon, there was a series of gems that I immediately took to heart and began planning for some future day when I could throw a dinner party of my own. First off, I liked that he mentioned the choosing of guests, saying that they should be "courtly people," people who will "enhance each other as persons."

If you feel uncomfortable about the idea of only inviting people you like to supper, consider this: In the everyday hospitality, you will have the Hubbles and the Johnsons at the same time, and the Johnsons, who are unbelievers, will require patience and care and hard conversational work. There should, as you are feeling, be plenty of times in life when you practice hospitality to people who require effort and aren't your favorite people.

But every once in a while, you should give a dinner where you just invite people who know and love each other, people you know and love. You should do it as a great gift to your guests and as a way of toeing into eternity. The feast is coming wherein we sit with people who have been united in their shared love of Christ. It will be dinner with friends.

In February of last year, I hosted my first dinner party that didn't rely on anyone else's house or cooking to pull off. I pulled out a favorite recipe book, *Barefoot in Paris*,[9] and resolved that the only rule for my menu was everything had to come from this book. Weeks in advance, I sorted and discussed the guest list with my husband.

"Not only do we want them to be people we like," I said, "we want them all to like each other."

I asked each couple to come dressed up, and I told the husbands that they'd be taking turns helping me to serve their wives each course. I borrowed a tablecloth and my mother's antique silverware, and spent time learning to fold napkins so they stand up. I asked a butcher to "french" my meat, which is when they clean off the bone that's sticking out, purely for presentation. I spent an hour making place cards. Yes indeed, the frivolity.

On the night of Valentine's Day, we had six places set. (One of our couples had to cancel due to illness! Flexibility, you see, even for your *convivium.*) The lighting was mostly candle. The guests brought little hostess gifts. The women were in heels. My husband wrote out his prayer ahead of time. We all pulled our chairs in, admired the matching dishware, and drank deep of sweet conversation and laughter. Our friends left with a verbal assumption that we'd do it again next year, and of course, they are right.

Do try this at home. Give yourself and your friends an occasion for rejoicing and resting in each other's company. Present an opportunity for each of you to remember that he is walking among kings and queens of both a present and future realm. True, we are poor in spirit, citizens of a far-off land and sojourners in the curse of creation, but we are also heirs who will someday judge angels. Occasionally, we should dress, gather, and eat as if this were true—

> On this mountain the LORD of hosts will make for all peoples
> a feast of rich food, a feast of well-aged wine,
> of rich food full of marrow, of aged wine well refined
> (Isaiah 25:6).

FOOD FOR THOUGHT

Discuss

- How often do you practice hospitality? What factors contribute to the frequency (or infrequency)?
- Do you tend to be better at the details of serving a meal, or at connecting with guests in a meaningful way around the meal?
- When was the last time you had a non-Christian in your home?

Practice

- Set up a schedule for practicing hospitality in your home. Start small, but challenge yourself. Every Friday? Every other Sunday? Once a month?
- It's helpful to have a "company meal"—something standard that you make whenever you have company. This means you don't have to think about the food so much; you can focus on getting people invited and then enjoying their company.
- Be prepared with cans, frozen goods, flour, and dried beans to feed more people than you expected with little notice. Your hospitality should be relaxed enough that another chair can always be pulled up.
- Plan a dinner party for good friends.

Read

- Dive into *The Gospel Comes with a House Key* by Rosaria Butterfield for a challenging proposal of hospitality as kingdom work.
- Read *Eve in Exile* by Rebekah Merkle for a rebuttal of feminism in America and a defense of homemaking as spiritual warfare.

CHAPTER 6

Learning to Cook

THE JOY OF DOING SOMETHING POORLY

I was 32 when I started cooking. Up until then, I just ate.

—JULIA CHILD

From Memory: 2018

I am 12 weeks along now. The sickness is subsiding, and I feel all God's mercy because others have it so much worse. My own mother was sick for the first five months of every pregnancy—seven of them. Others are sick the whole time.

I stand at the stove, and my three-year-old stands on a chair next to me. I'm sure this is crazy, but I'm letting her turn pieces of Cajun sausage in the pan. She tells me that when she's four, she'll be grown up enough to make food by herself, using the big pot. I tell her she's getting real close, real close.

She sits on the floor a few minutes later with a stalk of celery and a little cutting board. A butter knife is in her hand, after much negotiation over the steak knife she wanted to use. She's chopping the celery very slowly. When she's done, I'm going to let her throw it in the pot.

I remember that I like to cook—when I'm not dying of

hormone-induced nausea. Maybe I should try something new, like meatballs. Have I really never made meatballs?

Learning to Cook When It's Not Your Gifting

I didn't do much cooking as a kid or a young adult. When I was a kid, there were too many accidents when people tried to teach me. They let me make a cake one time, and I didn't put the oil in and didn't set a timer. I had a reputation for absentmindedness that was well earned by determined escapism into books and an inability to focus on tasks that weren't my idea. My sister once witnessed me walk into the kitchen, get a piece of bread, put it on the counter, open the fridge, and pour a cup of milk onto it. Then I snapped to attention and looked over at her with a strange "Where was I?" confusion on my face, and left the room.

The upshot was that I managed to evade the task of cooking well into adulthood. If other siblings came more naturally to the task, it was easier for everybody to let me off the hook. Occasionally, if I was allowed to "invent" a recipe, I got interested for a moment. For instance, I got fascinated with making dessert pasta for a while. At 12, I cooked a pound of fettuccine and drenched it with plain sugar and a chocolate sauce of my own devising (knowing nothing about chocolate, fettuccine, or sauce except that I liked each of them). What resulted was disgusting, and even I didn't try to eat it.

The dessert pasta fascination went dormant but was reawakened ten or so years later. As a young college graduate, I had friends over and made dessert lasagna. This time it was from a recipe online— a recipe that sounded logical enough to con me into buying a pile of rather expensive ingredients. It involved flat noodles boiled in sugar water, sweetened ricotta cheese, and layers of kiwi, blackberry, and strawberry. The concept was everything I ever wanted in a food—starchy, fruity, and a combination of two things every-body loves but never thought about combining (lasagna! dessert!).

My girlfriends, invited solely for the occasion of tasting this deli-cacy, sat around the table with enormous slabs on their plates. They dug in. About 60 seconds later, after a second bite to make sure I wasn't imagining it, I burst out with: "Oh no. This is terrible, isn't it?" Everyone laughed and pushed their plates away in relief. It *was* terrible. Inedibly so.

I came into marriage knowing how to make about half a dozen things, none of which could be combined to make one complete meal. I could make chicken tenderloin, bruschetta, scrambled eggs, jambalaya, box brownies, and my mother's recipe for wheat bread. These might sound like fancy things to only know how to make, but they followed a predictable line of items I'd been forced to learn at home (bread had been my job for about a year when I was 13) or become fascinated with long enough to make twice (really practi-cal stuff like bruschetta).

The things I had never made included: chocolate chip cookies, any kind of casserole, any kind of soup, meat loaf, anything with beans, any successful from-scratch dessert, spaghetti sauce, chicken pot pie, anything to bring to a church potluck. If I was ever forced to make something to serve somebody, it cost me a great deal of con-centrated thought and stressed second-guessing. I had no tricks, no shortcuts, no go-tos. Friends and coworkers generally understood that I was to be excused from the kitchen draft based on a preexist-ing condition.

My husband, thanks be to God, was not a foodie when we got married. He was a grateful eater who literally reached across and forked food off of other people's plates at supper ("Are you gonna eat that?" was one of the first questions he ever asked my sisters when he met them over a family meal).

But in our first little small-town apartment, with a Walmart as my sole source of groceries, I began to cook for two. I generally made dishes on the stove top—a pan-fried meat, usually chicken or pork, and a side vegetable in butter or oil. I'd do big veggie roasts in the oven that I ate over several days; I learned some soups that I would pack for lunch. Every evening meal began with a salad because I knew it might be the only vegetable my husband got for the day and because it made a weeknight meal feel like a real *event*.

I experimented with having people over but always felt awkward and self-conscious about the food. Nothing came naturally, and there was so much thought involved! Then we moved to a house with a smaller kitchen than the apartment and no dishwasher. I was in the kitchen more because of the dishwashing, but also I began cooking for a whole family as one daughter arrived and then another. Cooking for a family meant it was time to intentionally make enough to have leftovers. How else to feed people for lunch every day?

Learning to Bake

In 2016, I began to feel some kind of age-old, guttural urge calling to me from somewhere in my feminine subconscious. *Bake! Bake! It's time to bake!* All right, I said. Let's learn to bake. At Christmas, my husband heard me describe the call, and he and my in-laws bought me a Kitchenaid mixer. So, 2017 would be the year of bread, I decided.

I began with bagels in January. Bagels are a standard bread dough made with bread flour. They are boiled before baking. Endless topping combinations, endless delight in their chewy, fat bodies.

Then I opened my now-trusty *Betty Crocker Wedding Edition Cookbook*, opened to the quick breads, and began. I tried banana and zucchini breads, similar in concept to their autumn cousin, pumpkin bread. These are breads only in name—moist cakes that utilize the gooey properties of a fruit, vegetable, or squash, as the case may be. They are delicious, and they are impossible for anyone to really flub. Even me.

Then I tried more of the yeast breads, as the appetites presented themselves. I experimented with whole wheat breads and potato breads. I made my very first pizza dough from scratch. I got artisan sourdough lessons from a friend who goes through the entire three-day process every few weeks. I tried basic sandwich bread with varying mixtures of wheat and white flour. Sprouted breads and spelt breads and gluten-free breads. Ciabattas, waffles, sweet steakhouse rolls flavored with coffee and sorghum. Still on the to-do list: Croissants. Biscuits. Soft pretzels.

The thing that shocks me every time I bake is the magic of the process. Add just one more teaspoon of salt, and the result is different. Add an egg to an eggless dough, and it's a different dough. Use bread flour instead of all purpose, and you get the chewiness you crave. Feed that magic stuff—yeast—and it works and works, and its living activity brings you a kind of hocus-pocus result that you have to see to believe.

I think this is how I was won over to the structure of the recipe. When I was young, part of my problem was faulty logic—I believed that as long as all the ingredients went into the finished product, in any order, and were mixed around together, you should get the thing you set out to make. Pudding, angel-food cake, or any soup that contains onions would have proved me wrong. I should have taken a principle from math into the kitchen with me: Sometimes the order in which you add, multiply, divide, and subtract matters. This is elementary to solving math problems and elementary to cooking.

Sometimes you have to sauté the onions first. Sometimes you have to beat the egg whites alone.

But the golden, beautiful thing about it is that when you follow the recipe, you get the result in the picture. Usually.

Baking now reminds me of God's presence in physical matter, more so than any other cooking I may do. Perhaps it's because I always see it as a sort of miniature miracle, and "I am the bread of life" (John 6:35) is always just on the tip of my mind when I see the goodness of a risen loaf.

Jesus liked bread enough to compare himself to bread. Doesn't that surprise you a bit? It's surprising—just like the magic of rising dough is surprising. God is mixed up in all these magic reactions. He's responsible for the processes that wake up yeast, caramelize onions, and whip egg whites. He not only approves of our engagement in these things, but he's responsible for the fact that they keep working, time and time again.

The Sins of the Fathers

A few years ago, when I was working for the local paper, I started a Bible study for the women in the local jail. Ladies from my church and I went in on Monday nights and sang songs and read with the women. We were told early on that we weren't supposed to give Bibles to them to keep because they had copies already, and anyway they'd been caught tearing pages out and making cigarettes with them.

The most difficult thing about this ministry was trying to build relationships with the women outside the jail. It was easy to minister to them inside the four cinder-block walls of the meeting room—they had nowhere else to be. But as we took down notes about when each woman had scheduled court appearances, when each woman had been scheduled for parole, and whether she had a place to go, the real difficulties began to dawn on us. Many of the women had children somewhere in the community, being cared for by family or by the state. Many of them had not the means or desire to cut off relationships with the people who supplied them drugs—often boyfriends or husbands. Many of them showed enthusiasm for being placed in a halfway house or hosted by a family in our circle, but then made themselves scarce within a few days of getting released.

One of these women had children in a neighboring town. While she was still in the jail, she begged us to contact her mother-in-law and pick up the kids for church. I remember the first time I picked these kids up, driving down a difficult gravel driveway and knocking at several trailer doors before I found the right one. The children's grandmother answered, finally, and smoke exuded from the open door. The TV was on. Throughout the interior of the trailer, trash that mainly consisted of convenience food wrappers littered the floor and was piled on top of other miscellaneous items heaped onto every available floor space. A single footpath had been kept clear, a thread that connected the TV to the kitchen, the bathroom, and the door.

The two children were underdressed for an early spring day, I realized when we got outside. In the car, we blasted the heat, and they huddled under my jacket, and then at church we found blankets and sweaters for them. During the snack time between services, I rooted around in the kitchen and stole things from the potluck food to fill small plates and put those plates in front of the kids. They ate everything, and then cleaned plates again at lunch.

The hardest part of the day was dropping these kids off; a sinking feeling was always in my stomach as I watched them skip away toward the trailer. Eventually, the grandmother stopped taking our calls—she said the custody arrangement had changed, and it was too much trouble to keep up with which weekends they'd be available.

I've witnessed many other homes that reminded me of this one—most of them during the jail ministry years, or when I was selling subsidized insurance to people receiving disability. The same TV, on at any hour of the day; the same ubiquitous food wrappers by the couch, the same dinner table covered with enough paraphernalia that it was clearly never used. Recently, I read a description by British physician and writer Theodore Dalyrymple that sounded eerily familiar to what I'd seen in these homes.

Dalyrymple worked in a prison and in a hospital that was located in a rough British neighborhood. He often had doctors visiting from third-world countries to work and learn in the British hospital system, and he took them on tours of the neighborhood. The visitors remarked on the amount of trash piled in all of the yards and streets in front of this spacious, government-subsidized housing. *Does everyone eat fast food all the time here?* they wondered aloud.

Dalyrymple explained to them that in all his years visiting white households in the area, he'd never seen anyone cooking or taking meals together socially, "unless two people eating hamburgers together in the street as they walk along is counted as social."[1] Each individual in these homes ate whenever the urge came over them, so any opportunity to practice self-control in waiting for others was lost. "English meals," Dalyrymple observes, "are thus solitary, poor, nasty, brutish, and short."[2]

He then compares these poor, white British households to those run by Indian immigrants in the same area. The cultural difference is immense: Indians, he says, carefully purchase ingredients in local Indian stores and cook their communal meals. Dalyrymple concludes: "The willingness of Indians to take trouble over what they eat and to treat meals as important social occasions that impose obligations and at times require the subordination of personal desire is indicative of an entire attitude towards life that often permits them, despite their current low incomes, to advance up the social scale."[3]

This description is instructive to me because it's so familiar. I have experienced long periods—mostly as a single person living alone or as a guest in someone's home—of this lifestyle. I ate meals that were solitary, poor, nasty, brutish, and short—meals that were not "cooked" so much as "unwrapped" or "microwaved." These were meals that would wait for no man and that would have no real beginning, middle, or end because they were marked by nothing but stomach capacity and the length of a TV show. These were meals that served to underscore self-indulgence and to exacerbate loneliness, rather than to highlight service and foster relationship.

I know what it feels like to live this way; it's probably the reason these images have stuck with me so. A community table is such an important part of experiencing common grace in this world. It's such an important part of childhood. It's such an invaluable tool for loving and serving the unbeliever or the lonely Christian.

And, of course, it's important to recognize that there's no magic in the family table. Cooking and sitting down to eat together is not going to deliver saving gospel grace to anybody. Families have been eating together for thousands of years under the curse of sin, and the four corners of wood they sit around have been powerless to address their sickness of soul. Think of the desperate housewife in the 1950s, laying down perfectly appointed plates in front of father, sister, and brother and tucking a pint of whiskey into her apron. Think of the violent suppertime outbursts from dad witnessed by family across the world since the fall.

No, cooking and eating together has never fixed a single human heart.

I like to think of the family table instead as an opportunity. It won't deliver the gospel to anybody—but it's a *common grace* that God made available to mankind, like sunshine walks and covers on a bed, that bring comfort to tired bodies and minds. It won't deliver the gospel to anybody—but it's a *wise habit*, in terms of physical health and psychological health, a better alternative to the nasty and brutish private meal. It won't deliver the gospel to anybody—but it's an *opportunity for the gospel*, a place of meeting where your family culture can be developed and Scripture can be studied and sung, where parents and children can, if they care to, feed on more than just the food. It won't deliver the gospel to anybody—but it is *a way of procuring an audience for the gospel* among those who are strangers to you until you get them under your roof and feed them something.

Eating with somebody is an expression of intimacy. Intimacy is not the gospel, but it's a tool for advancing the gospel. Learning to cook—however simply—is something you can do with the kingdom of heaven as your goal. It's not just a way of illustrating something about the kingdom—the peace and joy of it, the bounty to be found in it, the self-giving service intrinsic to it. Cooking is also a practical means of advancing the kingdom through evangelism. When you keep a table, you are keeping an outpost of peace. You're defending something that is worth defending. You're protecting something good and beautiful.

And if you have kids, you're serving them in a way they will not understand until much later. You're providing a meeting place where the good things about a family can be practiced and enjoyed. You're putting in a scaffolding, a structure around which much more can be built, with potential for bodily, cultural, relational, and spiritual benefit.

I am, you can tell, a huge proponent of sitting down around a table every night. But I'm also aware of the sacrifice this requires—and I'm aware that in most cultures most of the sacrifice falls to mom. She's usually the one who decides what to feed people at that table. She's usually the one who has to add this to her long list of concerns for the day. She may be the one who has to push this vision uphill, against scheduling forces. She may be the one who has to choose the undignified tasks of meal preparation over and against other tasks to which she feels more suited. Statistically speaking, all of these things may end up being her responsibility, although they'll be immeasurably easier if a husband is present and on deck to make the family meal a priority.

But I can't think of any person who's responsible for other people that I wouldn't give this advice to: *It's worth it. It's worth your effort to make the community meal happen, if at all possible, when at all possible.*

If you don't have kids or family responsibilities, there are so many other ways you can take up responsibility for a community table. You can have regularly scheduled nights of home cooking for friends. You can invite yourself into other homes to share a meal, even if all you bring is a cake from the grocery. You can bring food to those who aren't able to get out, and share the table with them. The responsibility of holding the table is not just for stay-at-home moms or domestic goddesses; it's a lifelong opportunity available to anyone with access to a sink and a stove.

Cooking and the Eternal Soul

On the one hand, cooking brings you into the present and reminds you that you are only human. You may be an eternal soul; you may have an education; you may believe yourself to be made for all kinds of important destinies of your own devising, but in the end, you're a physical being with a belly and a couple of hands, and to use those two hands to knead and turn dough 50 times is really something. It's not a waste of time to engage with something physical that results in a physical product that will be (very soon) physically eaten up and dissolved.

You're humbling yourself when you condescend to soak beans in a pot for the seventh time this month. You're choosing to spend time on something that feels, for many of us, menial. Feeding ourselves or our families by hand is something we might have been taught is beneath us.

Also, if it's something we do regularly, it becomes a job. And like any other activity, you usually don't have as much fun with it after it becomes your job. But daily cooking is like other humble tasks in that, if we lean into them and do them as unto the Lord, they change us in good ways. Sweeping the floor and folding laundry can do this for you as well.

In some ways, the attitude with which you engage yourself in the menial is the truest measurement of your joy. I find it easier to exude joy during extreme circumstantial highs and extreme circumstantial lows. A trip, a job, or a baby can bring joy into even the most ungrateful heart. Crisis and loss produce tears, but when the loss can be categorized as "suffering" and is innocently come by, I often find it one of the easier times to reach for joy. The intensity of the experience is enough to put me on alert: *Now is the time to exhibit joy, because this is a blessing or a trial.*

It's the long seasons of middle ground that seem to me the most difficult testing ground for joy. And to me, cooking is a symbol of this ground. Feeding people again and again and again means you aren't going to be excited about it every time. It won't be romantic, and it may not be particularly challenging.

So if you come to the task with an attitude of superiority, the task will quickly remove your dignity from you. Dismembering a raw chicken brings with it a certain breakdown of exalted self-esteem. But if you come to the task as someone who knows herself to be dust

returning to dust, you won't have these startling moments of real-
ization: *How on earth did I get here, doing this every day? I was going
to be an actress.* Most everybody in history has been here, doing this
every day. That's what it means to be human.

On the other hand, the task of cooking can also be a bridge into
eternity, into the spiritual metaphors that Jesus himself used so
often. Knowing that his listeners were dust-people, hungry several
times a day and dependent on grain to stay alive, he promised to
give them what they needed: bread. So, he treated the physical needs
of the dust-body as a bridge to the eternal needs of the soul. As Jesus
spoke and worked, our dependence on food became a way of understanding our dependence on God himself. Jesus made something
clear to us: We have a much deeper need than our need for bread.
He started the conversation with food and ended it with himself.

Food was a constantly recurring metaphor that he reached for
again and again, as a dust-man talking to other dust-men: "Don't be
anxious about your life, what you will eat or what you will drink, or
about what you'll wear," he told the people during his most famous
sermon. "Have you noticed the birds? Your heavenly Father feeds
them; he'll feed you too. Seek first the kingdom of God and his
righteousness, and all these things will be added to you" (The exact
quote can be found in Matthew 6:25-26,33 in the Sermon on the
Mount).

He quoted Deuteronomy to Satan the tempter: "Man shall not
live by bread alone, but by every word that comes from the mouth
of God" (Deuteronomy 8:3, quoted in Matthew 4:4). And with
that, the tempter's desire was thwarted—the desire to see Jesus reach
for physical bread from some source besides faith. In Jesus's answer,
we see the spiritual problem beneath our gluttony and our food
laws too. We don't live by bread alone; our needs run to the Father
himself.

In John's Gospel, Jesus identified his own self as the bread needed to satisfy hunger forever:

> Truly, truly, I say to you, it was not Moses who gave you the bread from heaven, but my Father gives you the true bread from heaven. For the bread of God is he who comes down from heaven and gives life to the world.

> I am the bread of life; whoever comes to me shall not hunger, and whoever believes in me shall never thirst...Your fathers ate the manna in the wilderness, and they died. This is the bread that comes down from heaven, so that one may eat of it and not die. I am the living bread that came down from heaven. If anyone eats of this bread, he will live forever. And the bread that I will give for the life of the world is my flesh (John 6:32-33,35,49-51).

He had already said something similar to the woman at the well: "Everyone who drinks of this water will be thirsty again, but whoever drinks of the water that I will give him will never be thirsty again. The water that I will give him will become in him a spring of water welling up to eternal life" (John 4:13-14).

Jesus clearly returned to this gospel presentation again and again. He fed the people physically, and then explained that he was going to feed them spiritually. He stood at the watercooler and explained that he was the water that would well up into eternal life. He observed the neediness of hungry birds and then connected it directly to hungry children with a bounteous Father.

If he was willing to present good news in this way again and again, we can follow his example again and again. We feed people, but we never believe the lie that their physical needs are everything. They may believe this lie, but we can use their physical needs as a bridge to their spiritual ones. We do the same thing for ourselves, preaching the good news of bread broken for us even as we bow our heads over physical bread. We do the same thing for our children, feeding their little bodies to show them what good fathers might do, and then telling them about the Father who feeds souls. Food was an evangelistic bridge that Jesus walked over again and again. We can use it the same way in our humble kitchens with our humble pots and pans.

FOOD FOR THOUGHT

Discuss

- Do you feel personally humbled by cooking, by the messiness and the monotony of it?

- Do you feel personally dignified by cooking, by the ritual and the metaphor of it?

- Why do you think Jesus used food as an evangelical tool, connecting with people over meals, physically feeding people via miracles, and using food in his parables?

Practice

- If possible, find a way to get your family together for meals. Consider cutting back on commitments to prioritize it. With teenagers, consider asking them to commit to one or two days a week, to avoid scheduling things on those nights.

- Try baking bread—real bread with yeast. (Look up recipes on the King Arthur Flour website for a real education in baking. They have whole pages on basic things like "How to Measure Flour" that will amaze you.)

- See if you can figure out the dessert pasta thing; maybe you'll succeed where I failed.

Read

- Luxuriate in *My Life in France* by Julia Child, with descriptions that will make you terribly excited about learning to cook.[4]

- Read *Life at the Bottom* by Theodore Dalyrmple for a revealing description of an entire culture, including the shortsighted vision that makes no time for family meals.

CHAPTER 7

The Mirror

FOOD AND BODY IMAGE

I was conscious, as only a very young girl can be, of the fact that I
did not have the looks of my aunts or my beautiful mother. I was
the ugly duckling. I had such an intense longing for approval and
love that it forced me to acquire self-discipline.

—ELEANOR ROOSEVELT[1]

From Memory: 2003

I am standing on the scale in the Hermitage YMCA. It's one of those
that you see in doctor's offices with sliding metal pieces that offer
a precise, balanced measurement. I've been to two workout classes
already this morning. I mentally subtract a few of the pounds in
front of me to account for a full water bottle I drank during those
classes.

Either way, the scale is showing a number that is not satisfac-
tory. I don't know why the number won't go down. I'm doing all the
right things. I pull out a food diary from a workout bag that smells
of damp towels and look at yesterday's entry:

- 1 piece wheat bread—100 calories
- 1 pat of butter—50 calories

- 2 apples—120 calories
- 1 piece chicken—150 calories
- Brown rice—100 calories
- 1 apple—120 calories
- 1 piece chocolate—60 calories
- Total—700 calories

So nice and low! I'll have to tell Adrienne, my dieting partner. But then I flip to the day before that. The total is 1,500 calories. And the day before that was 1,800. Our goal right now is around 1,100. So that's why. One day of 600 won't cut it. But a few days might.

The seniors start to file in after their 9 a.m. water aerobics class. They sit on benches in the locker room around me and start to undress. Skin hangs from their arms as they strip swimsuits off, unselfconsciously revealing breasts and bottoms for a few seconds while they locate dry garments.

They talk about kidneys. They talk about second opinions and blood-pressure medications. They talk about their husbands, who are sitting in the lobby already, drinking coffee at round metal tables. What they don't talk about at any point is calories. For them, the cares of the body have shifted. No longer are they worried about waistlines—now the organs inside their waistlines are struggling in active duty. It seems impossible to me that I'll ever be like them.

I walk out on slightly unsteady limbs, feeling pleasantly empty and resolving to post some of those pictures I cut out of a *Shape* magazine on my bedroom wall for extra motivation. If I could see into the future, I would see 25 pounds gained over the next three years, and a new habit of purging to accompany inevitable binges. I would see years of dominating behavior and a body that will never do what I so desperately, desperately wanted it to do. I would see years of failure and lost time. But even if I saw it all clearly in front of me, I'd still respond by opening another diet magazine and setting a new goal and resolving to attend another cardio kickboxing class. Even knowing the future, I would have simply tried to avert it—tried to avert it by continuing the chase.

If I could see further into the future, I'd see aging organs shutting down and strength slowly failing over time. I'd see a death of some kind coming for me. But I can't see into the future. All I can see is a mirror.

America and the Fear of Pleasure

In the late 1800s, Wilbur Olin Atwater was a scientist on a mission. He was the person who brought basic macronutrients to the American awareness, along with the calorie—a measure of the energy obtained from foods in the form of heat generated. He received a special assignment from the USDA to study the calorie in 1893, using metal respiratory chambers and other strange contraptions.

His mission was not just to understand the calorie, but to transform the American eater into someone who sees food as fuel, not as a source of pleasure. Americans were eating too much fat and too much starch, he declared in an article in 1892, and they were short on lean protein. They were also eating too much in general, he said, and "how much harm is done to health by our one-sided and excessive diet, no one can say."[2]

In an 1895 USDA publication, Wilbur wrote:

> In our actual practice of eating we are apt to be influenced too much by taste, that is, by the dictates of the palate...We need to observe our diet and its effects more carefully, and regulate appetite by reason...Part of the principle is found in the fact that the human body is a machine.[3]

Around this time, women began to join a movement to bring the domestic arts into a new era: the era of science. These women saw their jobs not only as moral guides and domestic nurturers, but as engineers for the good of household health. Ellen Richards wrote in her 1885 book *Food Materials and Their Adulterations,*

> Strong men and women cannot be "raised" on insufficient food. Good-tempered, temperate, highly moral men cannot be expected from a race which eats badly cooked food, irritating to the digestive organs and unsatisfying to the appetite. Wholesome and palatable food is the first step in good morals, and is conducive to ability in business, skill in trade, and healthy tone in literature.[4]

So good food leads to good literature, and bad food...well, you know where I'm going. I wonder if this explains the *Twilight* series?

This attitude about food as fuel is so common that I bet you've heard someone say it or read it in a diet book. It overlooks a basic fact about people that will always come back to bite us: We're not machines, and food has more purposes than to fuel our mechanical bodies. When we turn our kitchens into labs and attempt to live as machines without tastes, we'll find ourselves going against the grain of the way we were made, as well as thumbing our nose at the substances God made in such varied abundance. As Michelle Stacy grimly commented, "This is the sort of outlook that might lead to a firm belief in yogurt and ricotta, mixed with cornstarch, as a dead ringer for cream sauce."[5]

It's just not so. Food is more than fuel. The body is more than a machine. And yogurt and ricotta, mixed with cornstarch, will never taste like cream sauce. But America's distrust of pleasurable food has been with us for a long time. It's how you end up with a nation of gluttonous but guilty people who firmly believe if they were more virtuous, they'd resist the pleasures of food permanently and reach their full potential.

Food and the Shape of Us

For most of the women I know, food and appearance are inextricably tied. We have been swimming in this environment for our entire lives. We may not know the history of America and food, and we may be dimly aware that other cultures approach food differently. And we all see the same headlines about disease and obesity—this is old news.

Sociologists and scientists connect the global rise in body weight to industrial farming, which has allowed core crops like wheat, corn, and rice to be produced on a regulated and massively successful scale. Our global culture has made a trade. We've got more and cheaper food for most of the people alive today, with starvation no longer the primary concern of most ordinary families everywhere. But admittedly, we have some new problems we've never faced before.

In the US, corn is supplying most of the calories that turn into most of the fat that is hanging around on most of our bodies. It's a subsidized crop, and one that is grown on almost a hundred million acres of land out in the American corn belt. The number of calories we obtain from corn is not what you'd guess. You might look at your cob and tortilla intake and think corn isn't a big part of your life, but as writer Michael Pollan points out in describing his family's McDonald's meal:

> I figure my 4-ounce burger, for instance, represents nearly 2 pounds of corn (based on a cow's feed conversion rate of 7 pounds of corn for every 1 pound of gain, half of which is edible meat). The nuggets are a little harder to translate into corn, since there's no telling how much actual chicken goes into a nugget; but if 6 nuggets

contain a quarter pound of meat, that would have taken a chicken half a pound of feed corn to grow. A 32-ounce soda contains 86 grams of high-fructose corn syrup (as does a double-thick shake), which can be refined from a third of a pound of corn; so our three drinks used another one pound. Subtotal: 6 pounds of corn.[6]

The nutritional value of our food is changing, and everyone has already told us about it. Food that derives all its charm from fat, salt, and sugar is not doing any of us any favors. But the condition of the food industry is such that for every last one of us, it takes more effort and money to avoid these things than to live off of them. That's why, statistically speaking, the poorer the American, the fatter the American, and the more likely we are to get most of our calories from these sources.

It may be a lifestyle choice, but it's a choice that has been thrust on every one of us from birth for the last 50 or so years, and one that our great-grandmothers escaped. They worked hard for their food, but they didn't have to work hard for food and also constantly resist very attractive tastes available literally everywhere, at cut-rate prices, all while struggling to maintain the bodies of Brazilian warrior princesses.

As Christian women, we don't need to spend a lot of time figuring out who is to blame for this state of affairs. How we got here has to do with complicated economics and complicated sin as well. But it's helpful to remember that as we struggle through battles with the scale, we no longer have to worry about scrounging up enough food to keep our children alive. This has been the first question of food for most of history.

A thousand years ago, most of the human lifetime was taken up with the business of getting enough food and cooking it. This is still the case in some areas of the world. Take food historian Rachel

Laudan's description of hand-grinding grain, something that house-
wives and servants have been doing for millennia:

> Grinding may look easy, and it is, for the first ten min-
> utes. To grind a quantity of grain, though, as I found out
> when I tried, takes skill, control, physical strength, and
> time. I was quickly panting, sweaty, and dizzy, my hair
> in my eyes, and the [grinding stone] slipping at awk-
> ward angles. Grinding is hard on the knees, hips, back,
> shoulders, and elbows, causing arthritis and bone dam-
> age...Even today Mexican women in remote villages
> grind five hours daily to prepare enough maize for a fam-
> ily of five or six.[7]

I don't bring this up to take us on a guilt trip of the "finish your
plate because children are starving in China" variety. I bring it up to
say that our struggles are struggles of stewardship. Remembering
the very different struggles of other people can give us fresh perspective on the struggles we ourselves have been assigned by our Father.

Because the thing is, no matter what we do, and unless we are
called to go to the mission field in very specific regions of the world,
we will not be in this position of grinding five hours a day to feed
our families. We have different challenges to face. Our challenges
have to do with decisions, with images, with self-control, with generosity, and with resources. In a word, ours are the challenges of
stewardship.

So, knowing this, what do we do with our body battles? How
can we be faithful under these circumstances? How can we be truth-
ful in the face of these particular lies? Where, as women of the
Lord, do we thrust these thoughts about thighs and love handles
and stretch marks? How can we be grateful women? How can we
fight the world, the flesh, and the devil instead of getting mired

in a disappointing fight against negative self-talk and vending machines? How can our voices be voices of peace, life, and sanity in a world that shouts constant conflicting messages to us and our fellow women? They want us to be disciplined *and* self-indulgent! Thin *and* proud of being fat! Shamelessly provocative *and* independent of the male eye! Weak, so weak that we spend a lot of time telling each other how needy we are, and also stronger than even we can comprehend!

Instead, we have a Father who asks us to hide ourselves in him, to be obedient even when our exterior circumstances aren't glamorous. He asks us to be courageous and to take up crosses. He asks us to be adorned with a character of humility and gentleness. Our bodies are instruments to be used for righteousness, come to find out—and the world can't understand why our bodies keep getting used for advertising.

The Message We Want or the Message That Gives Life

Even in the church, sometimes, Christian women get a sort of trickled-down word from Oprah. The Christianized version of "you are woman; you could be an underwear model; you are *enough!*" is a repeated refrain of "God made you beautiful, and it's time for you to believe that hard enough to stop feeling insecure about yourself."

I remember packing this very message up in a suitcase and carrying it to Northern Ireland to share it with a group of Irish teen girls on a mission trip when I was in college. The teen girls in this small town we went to were all what you call "high risk." Many of them smoked at the age of 10 or 12, were sexually active around the same time, and snuck bottles of vodka into the sleepovers we hosted for them.

One of the exercises we set up was a mirror on a table, where they were supposed to sit down, look at themselves, and say the first thing that came to mind. The first thing that came to mind was inevitably negative and critical. Then we asked them to come up with three things they saw that they liked. *Yes*, we would say. *God made you; you should be able to appreciate what he made. Isn't what he made beautiful?*

In the process of trying to bring the gospel to these girls, we had no better idea than plunking them down in front of a mirror to get higher doses of the self they were already sick of. They were busy stifling the strong pain of young life with sex and drugs and eating disorders, and our bright idea was to make them do self-affirmations.

What will a 12-year-old girl who hates her life see in the mirror? She'll see an image she hates but is stuck with. She'll see the person she is more dedicated to serving than anyone else: herself. She's serving herself poorly, but it's the self that she's most concerned about protecting from pain, making comfortable and happy, exalting to importance if at all possible. The mirror is the last thing she needs. What she needs is to peer at an image of Christ and see what worth looks like. She needs to be reminded that God made her on purpose—yes—but this message of handiwork isn't good news until she is told that what he made is being marred and destroyed by sin and death and that his intention is to remake her into the image of Christ.

The beauty she seeks is about so much more than noses and ears, Irish freckles and soft, white hips. It's about loves and hates, motives and thoughts, joys and tasks. He can make that kind of beauty in her, but sitting in front of a mirror until the beauty shows up isn't going to help anybody. Her eyes need to be drawn away from herself. "If anyone would come after me," Jesus tells her, "let [her] deny herself and take up [her] cross and follow me" (Matthew 16:24).

And we grown women in good churches are sometimes prone to feed each other the same messages that were so unhelpful to these Irish teens. We insist to one another, again and again, that each other is beautiful. We contend with the lies of Satan—real lies about worthlessness or the grossness of bodies or the hopelessness of life in the trenches—but we contend with these lies using dull weapons. "God made you, and that means you're worthy and beautiful," we tell each other. Sometimes we attend conferences so we can hear "You are fearfully and wonderfully made" spoken over and over again to us using different words. Sometimes we get online and give each other compliments about our beautiful postpartum bodies or our photogenic faces.

But if we remain with our noses glued to a mirror, we'll never get the feeling of security we're looking for. The words of our kind and well-meaning sisters will be powerless to combat the lies of the enemy.

What we need is transformation. And that transformation comes in only one way: "And we all, with unveiled face, beholding the glory of the Lord, are being transformed into the same image from one degree of glory to another. For this comes from the Lord who is the Spirit" (2 Corinthians 3:18).

We are transformed only by gazing on him. When we see his suffering, his faithfulness, his wisdom, his high priesthood, his sonship, his promises fulfilled—in a word, his glory—we become transformed into beings who are also glorious. Perfect like our Father is perfect—that's where we're headed. And the only way to head there is to fill our eyes not with ourselves but with the One who "in every respect has been tempted as we are, yet without sin. Let us then with confidence draw near to the throne of grace, that we may receive mercy and find grace to help in time of need" (Hebrews 4:15-16).

We have a real problem, and Jesus is the real person who is both powerful enough to address our problem and empathetic enough to be approached with it.

Our longing to be made gorgeous is actually not all made up of vanity and a steady diet of foolish advertising. Our longing to be made gorgeous is motivated by a deep and legitimate ache to see something wrong being made right. We're dissatisfied with the parts of us we believe to be lacking in glory, to be shameful in some way, and that feeling comes from a place in our hearts that is still reeling from the fall and still longing to be restored.

The world thinks that shame is constructed and that putting plus-sized women on billboards in their underwear is going to remove shame from all of us. But we know shame is so deeply rooted it can't be done away with so easily. We know it's not a matter of perception. Satan isn't working with purely fabricated material when he tells us we're worth nothing because our backs jiggle and we keep buying cookies. He's working with the materials of truth and twisting them before he feeds them to us: Something *is* wrong with us, but that something goes much deeper than jiggling backs. And far from being hopelessly beyond help or being capable of helping ourselves with a gym membership and a campaign against body shaming, God is both able and willing to change us from the root upward.

Not only can we be free of all this jiggling-back, self-hatred nonsense, we can be daughters and workers in a kingdom that (thank goodness) is not about us at all. It's about God, the glorious Father who adopts and transforms. It's a kingdom of people laying down their lives for one another as they follow the example of the One who broke death by laying down his life for his enemies. There isn't a billboard in sight. There's only Christ.

Death and Body Image

I'm in my thirties now. I see things in the mirror I never saw before—dry skin and wrinkles, weirdly frizzy hair. During my last pregnancy, I got varicose veins for the first time. They ache and give me a sinking feeling of decay when I crane my head around to look at the back of my right knee in the shower. I also have recently had issues with bruising—something about an unexplained short-age of platelets that may or may not be caused by an autoimmune disorder.

I'm dying. That's the long and short of it. I begin to under-stand what the older folks have tried to explain to me before: Aging comes for you without your consent. You still feel like a sprightly girl of 15, attending one exercise class after another and bouncing back overnight from the flu. But when you wake up in the morning and trudge to the bathroom, you realize you're not 15 anymore, and you'll never be 15 again. In fact, the only thing you know for sure is that you're on a train of death, and it's steadily bringing you closer to something you didn't choose. You are dying. Nobody asked you if it was okay with you. Nobody promised you anything, except that your days are like grass, and you flourish "like a flower of the field; for the wind passes over it, and it is gone" (Psalm 103:15-16).

The only good news you can possibly hear, given the state of things, is that you don't need to be surprised about death. Your outer self is wasting away, but your spirit is being renewed day by day (2 Corinthians 4:16). When you watch spiritual maturity develop, and you see that your spirit is, in fact, being renewed day by day, it gives you yet another reason to expect death and cling to future life.

Then, too, you can look at the same passages that promise death and see the promises behind these promises. In Psalm 103, where we find pessimistic and disheartening descriptions for man—like "dust" and "grass"—we also see our very reason for life-giving hope. Our Father is tenderly leading us to newness and long life, even as our bodies fall apart:

> As a father shows compassion to his children,
>> so the LORD shows compassion to those who fear him.
> For he knows our frame;
>> he remembers that we are dust.
> As for man, his days are like grass;
>> he flourishes like a flower of the field;
> for the wind passes over it, and it is gone,
>> and its place knows it no more.
> But the steadfast love of the LORD is from everlasting to
>> everlasting on those who fear him,
>> and his righteousness to children's children,
> to those who keep his covenant
>> and remember to do his commandments.
> The LORD has established his throne in the heavens,
>> and his kingdom rules over all (Psalm 103:13-19).

Yes, our bodies are like grass, but the steadfast love of the Lord is from everlasting to everlasting on those who fear him. Yes, our bodies are dust, but the Lord has established his throne in the heavens, and this throne is the thing we set our eyes on as we watch time pull our dust back to dust.

Our bodies aren't a good place to put all our investment money. Even if we manage to wrestle them into shape when we're young, and make it into middle and advanced age with some kind of dignified imitation of youth, we'll still have death to contend with. Our days are still like grass, even if we don't end up sitting naked around the YMCA locker room with flapping arms talking about kidneys with our girlfriends.

But God our Father knows our frame and is tenderly, compassionately leading us through the valleys of the shadow of death. These valleys include pulling on pants two weeks after giving birth, when the stitches come out. They include biopsies and mammograms.

They include the stockings you have to wear for varicose veins. We shall fear no evil. For he is with us.

The Sin Behind the Sin

Sometimes our preoccupation with body image can blind us to the spiritual battles we engage in. It's a thought I've had often since my intensive days of battling bulimia. People who are dealing with one difficult-to-conquer sin of the flesh with addictive properties—like pornography or gluttony or alcoholism—tend to start approaching the issue as if it is the only problem they have. It is scary, so they give it their full attention because they see that it's going to eat them alive.

But eventually, they may fight it so hard and for so long that they don't understand how many ordinary sins stand behind their Big Bad Sin. Laziness, vanity, pride, relational immaturity, and resentment may be standing behind and motivating their Big Bad Sin, but they can only see the porn. They assume that when the porn is gone, the battle will be over. But what they don't realize is that Christians of every kind are fighting sin all the time. The Big Bad Sin has stunted their growth by keeping them ignorant of the other sins that needed fighting. They didn't know the sin of worry—though unglamorous and ordinary, and something that almost every Christian has to deal with—was there all along, still waiting to be addressed, and contributing to the Big Bad Sin as well.

What stands behind our obsession with bodily appearance? Here are some potential sins-behind-the-sin, but you may, on closer examination, see others.

- **Fear of man** (Galatians 1:10—"For am I now seeking the approval of man, or of God?...If I were still trying to please man, I would not be a servant of Christ.")

- **Idolatry** (Isaiah 42:8; Matthew 6:21—"For where your treasure is, there your heart will be also.")

- **Lack of self-control** (Deuteronomy 21:20; 1 Corinthians 6:12-20, here 6:12—"'All things are lawful for me,' but not all things are helpful. 'All things are lawful for me,' but I will not be dominated by anything.")

- **Pride** (James 4:6—"God opposes the proud but gives grace to the humble.")

- **Vanity** (Proverbs 31:30—"Charm is deceitful, and beauty is vain, but a woman who fears the LORD is to be praised.")

- **Laziness** (Proverbs 23:21—"For the drunkard and the glutton will come to poverty, and slumber will clothe them with rags.")

- **Lack of love** (Romans 12:9-21, here 12:9-10—"Let love be genuine. Abhor what is evil; hold fast to what is good. Love one another with brotherly affection. Outdo one another in showing honor.")

You may think the food, or the magazines, or the scale are your biggest problem. But perhaps your greater problem is laziness—you don't want to do the laundry, so you're eating to avoid doing laundry. Perhaps your problem is fear of man—you worry about what your mom will say if she sees you've gained a few pounds. Perhaps your problem is pride—you desire to be powerful, and food is what you try to use to be in control. Perhaps your problem is lack of self-control—you want to give in to your own impulses and not experience the consequences. Perhaps your problem is vanity—far from having "low self-esteem," you're simply driven to be the best-looking woman in a room because this is where you get your confidence.

Seek to address the sin behind the sin, and you'll begin to understand the nature of your body-image struggles more clearly.

Another Weapon in the Battle

The Maudsley method, also called Family Based Treatment, was developed in the 1980s in a London hospital. It was developed as an outpatient treatment for anorexia nervosa in adolescents, and the core of the treatment is the family table.

In the Maudsley method, parents eat three meals a day and two snacks with their undernourished teenager. Many parents take a leave of absence from work in order to undertake this therapy. During the painful first phase, the unwilling young person is given no choice but to sit with the family and eat everything given to them; the first phase is primarily about weight gain. Typically, the young woman is at her angriest and most depressed during this phase, but parents are encouraged to keep up the family meals and the calories until the "refeeding" is complete, and she is no longer in a state of starvation. The "why" of the anorexia can be better addressed when her brain and body aren't starving to death.

This treatment, though stressful to the whole family and involving great inconvenience to parents, is demonstrably more successful than hospital stays and treatment centers (an 80 percent recovery rate is quite high for anorexia nervosa). It's interesting to observe that in many of these households, three family meals a day is a previously unheard-of concept. And to the private, obsessive inner life of the anorexic girl, family meals—however unpleasant to her—are a paradigm-shifting part of the process of recovery.

The power of treating food as a community endeavor shouldn't be overlooked as we seek to shake our more obsessive attitudes toward food and the body. We know our eyes need to be on Christ. But with our eyes on Christ, our hands are usually in something too. And it won't hurt us to examine the habits of our lives that can help us grow into women who are less absorbed with the mirror and the scale.

Food issues—diet obsession, overeating, etc.—are often characterized by private and even secret behavior. The binge or purge usually occurs in the privacy of one's home, without witnesses. The extreme diet is usually carried out in one person's head, observed on an individual basis. Even women who are in charge of feeding their families often diet alone, fixing a meal for themselves and a separate meal for their children and husbands. Isolation and separation usually accompany the quest for thinness. So, conversely, reorienting yourself to the community and family aspects of eating is one way of fighting your private, self-centered obsessions.

Do you have a family you cook for? Cook for everybody all at once. If you're trying to be healthy, find ways of cooking things for the whole family that promote wellness and enjoyment all around. (Stumped? Start with beans. Find out how to cook beans in ways you all enjoy, and you'll solve budget, diet, and *how-can-I-fill-up-all-these-people?* problems all at once.) If veggies are good for you, they're good for them too. If excessive sugar at every meal is bad for you, it's bad for them too. But it would be hard for you to maintain no-carbs-ever for the entire family—and maybe that's a good sign you shouldn't be trying it yourself.

And if you aren't feeding a family—single, married without children, or in the empty-nest years—there are still lots of ways to make food into a community practice. I have now been enjoying church potlucks every Sunday for ten years. The potluck means we eat a lot of things we wouldn't cook for ourselves, and it means we get to share table fellowship with our brothers and sisters so regularly that we actually know each other. It means we have to elbow around gently, being gracious about so-and-so's recipe for sugar-free, gluten-free dessert, as well as so-and-so's habit of always bringing white bread PB&J for the kids. It means we have to serve one another.

Another great ministry of the church is one in which anybody who is sick or has a new baby gets weeks of meals delivered to them by fellow church members. It takes a little bit of organization (easy with websites like takethemameal.com) and everybody pitching in. But it's a wonderful opportunity for rube cooks (like myself when I was single) to take a stab at cooking for other people's needs.

Also, aside from church-organized events, a person without family-feeding responsibilities can engage with community food in all kinds of personal ways. For instance, a young single man in our congregation who loves to cook often invites himself over to cook for families in the church. There are always aging people or people with disabilities in your community who live alone or in nursing homes and would welcome the chance to share a meal with someone else. Take them lunch, and eat it with them! Invite your single friends to supper, and form a little family meal of your own! Practice feeding other people and being fed by them!

Food is so much more than private enjoyment or private torture. It's an opportunity to love and serve others. And when you've got your hands busy in the mechanics of feeding people besides yourself, you've got something working for you instead of against you in the fight against diet obsession.

Fighting Worship with Worship

So, are you growing as a Christian? Are you taking advantage of the means of grace? Treating food as the Big Bad Sin will at some point only distract you from the spiritual growth that you should be attending to. The thing about human beings is that we need something to care about. If the tendency of your mind and heart is to pull back into gluttony or a new diet-of-the-week, the problem might be that you simply haven't exchanged pursuits. You are pursuing something with all your might, but your energy is being spent after wind.

You are a worshiper. Your impulse to worship and to run after something isn't going to go away. Perhaps your worship of food is only persisting because you refuse to see your halfheartedness in pursuing intimacy with Christ.

Do you have spiritual disciplines in place that will bring you into his presence via the Word and prayer on a daily basis? Are you engaged in your church as a servant who makes herself available to other believers and to the ministries of the church? Are you watching other Christian women to imitate their godliness and fervency, or are you watching them to imitate their style of dress, the cleanliness of their home, or their childrearing or workplace successes?

The thing is, your heart is a pursuing heart. It's running after something at all times; you are full of longings. So which lesser longings are you allowing to dim your longing for God? Which longings, pursued, are giving you a sensation of temporary fullness, allowing you to forever neglect your hunger for him?

The godliness quest cannot be happily combined with the thinness quest. The eyes are either on Christ or on the scale, but they can't be fully turned on both. This is not to say you can't think about physical matter without "breaking your concentration" on Christ. But there is a certain way of attending to the body that displaces our worship—because it *is* worship.

You keep asking—*How can I stop overeating and lose this weight?* Or even, *How can I stop worshiping food and the body?* But perhaps these are the wrong questions. Perhaps you're still fighting battles with a peripheral opponent. Your real problem is not hunger for food; your problem is a low appetite for God. Maybe you haven't applied yourself to the private, quiet practices that Christians have used to get to know him for millennia. Your attempts to rein in the chocolate habit—even in the name of Spirit-borne self-control—may be successful, but they'll only allow you to exchange idols for idols until your heart is in pursuit of the thing it was made to pursue.

FOOD FOR THOUGHT

Discuss

- What are some "sins behind the sin" that might be lurking behind your struggles with food and body image? Fear of man, idolatry, lack of self-control, pride, vanity, laziness, lack of love, or something else?

- Is death something you push out of your mind? Do you have a robust understanding of death as an unwelcome but ultimately defeated enemy? When you see signs of aging, for instance, do you think "wrinkle cream," or do you think "heaven"?

Practice

- Practice some ways of serving others with food. Take food to a family in medical crisis, or to a mom who just had a baby. Take food to shut-ins in your church or community, and sit down to eat it with them. Get your eyes off the scale and onto somebody with needs to be met.

- Assess yourself as a disciple of Christ: Are you taking advantage of the means of grace? Do you experience delight in and longing for the person of Jesus Christ? Are you regularly reading God's Word and engaging in prayer? Are you faithfully serving your church body and showing up to worship and hear the Word preached? If you aren't engaged in active pursuit of obedience, something will rush in to fill the space left.

Read

- Check out *Redeemed from the Pit* by Marie Notcheva, one of several good Christian counseling resources on eating disorders.[8]

- Read *Remember Death* by Matthew McCullough for a reminder that we aren't as familiar with death as previous generations have been, and an application of gospel hope to the fear of death we subconsciously carry.[9]

CHAPTER 8

Wine O'Clock

ALCOHOL AND THE CHRISTIAN WOMAN

"All things are lawful," but not all things are helpful. "All things are lawful," but not all things build up.

—1 CORINTHIANS 10:23

From Memory: 2018

I'm sitting in my friend's yard on a warm summer evening. Her house is on a hilltop surrounded by woods and one lone, neighboring farmhouse. Her garden is full of ripe produce, just a few hundred yards from where I sit. The little folding table has been covered with a tablecloth and set carefully with glasses, plates, silverware, and cloth napkins that I was in charge of folding but couldn't get to stand upright.

Dusk is just setting in, and five of us are pulling folding chairs in close around the table. Our kids are home with their fathers. We have copies of G.K. Chesterton's *Orthodoxy* tucked beside our plates, but we've determined we're going to eat first and then adjourn to the couches inside to discuss our chapters.

Our glasses are full of deep-red Syrah from California. The one among us who knows about wine has taken us through the steps of tasting to see if we can detect the pine needle and lavender notes.

We're supposed to able to detect a "chalky" finish, too, according to the wine guide. But I don't know that I do. All I know is it's a very nice wine, and I'm enjoying it. Many of us are on a second glass, a white, by the time we sit down to our meal.

The host has given us a traditional shrimp and grits dish as the main course. The grits are coarse grain, and whatever anybody says, the novelty of the large lumps of corn contributes to my enjoyment of the meal. It's gorgeous, the way shrimp and grits combine with good dairy to satisfy the human desire for protein, carbs, and fat.

Conversation is warm and hilarious. We are the Hartsville Literary Club, and something of a food club as well because when we have our meetings, there is often food and wine or food and tea. But the books are sustaining the conversation, and they're keeping us from getting stuck in the familiar ruts of domestic tips and stories about our children. We want an opportunity to exercise dormant parts of our minds and hearts, and these evenings are blessed opportunities to do just that.

For an hour on the lawn, we are tasting the company of fellow queens and pilgrims in pursuit of heaven. The wine is an agent of plenty and conviviality; it combines with the light and the written mental fodder and the grits to elevate us and remind us of what we're here for. We're courtiers in a kingdom that has yet to come. Our cheeks are warm and our spirits are buoyant, but everyone is in her right and clear mind. Our tongues are loosened but not to foolishness, and our moods are relaxed but not to oblivion. It is an oasis and a resting place, an evening's worth of sisterly fellowship that promises richer fellowship to come in another time and place.

A Moderationist Point of View

When it comes to drinking alcoholic beverages, I am a moderationist, which means that I find freedom in Scripture to partake moderately of alcohol. I don't plan to spend too much time in this chapter defending this position, mainly because I am writing primarily for other moderationist women who probably share my opinion about these matters. However, I will briefly lay out my position for clarity's sake, not so much to win any converts as to explain my own practice and rationale.

First of all, I think it's useful for each of us to remember we live in a particular context, and whatever else we know, we know our feelings and convictions are deeply affected by that context. I am influenced by the fact that I was not raised by alcoholics. A person who was raised by alcoholics would have a very different perspective. I am influenced by the fact that I'm in a rural area, where the majority of churches take a very dark view of alcohol, and people are afraid to go to the liquor store on the main highway because their cars will be recognized. I'm also influenced by the fact that I'm in a Baptist church, and the Baptists as a group have carried the prohibitionist torch for 200 years or so, originally responding to drunkenness and debauchery in the nineteenth century. I'm further influenced by the fact I run in primarily Reformed circles, which tend to be very open to moderate drinking for Christians.

In addition to our various contexts, we all have different fleshly habits as well. Some of us still smell the inside of a bar when a bottle of beer is cracked open. Some of us have bodies that taste the first sip and react like sharks when blood hits the water. Some of us hear the sound of fizz in the glass and think immediately of wild dancing, of dark rooms, of illicit encounters.

I acknowledge that it is almost impossible to approach the alcohol question without being heavily influenced by these personal experiences and by the culture in which you find yourself. So, as I defend my position here, I want to do so with a light touch, in the knowledge that others look at Scripture and draw a different conclusion.

The Bible speaks positively of alcohol consumption.

The first reason I feel freedom to partake of alcohol moderately is that I see this practice very positively described in Scripture. An early example in the Old Testament is Deuteronomy 14:24-27, in which God commands the Israelites about tithing. He gives them one payment option that surprises me:

> If the way is too long for you, so that you are not able to carry the tithe, when the LORD your God blesses you...then you shall turn it into money and bind up the money in your hand and go to the place that the LORD your God chooses and spend the money for whatever you desire—oxen or sheep or wine or strong drink, whatever your appetite craves. And you shall eat there before the LORD your God and rejoice, you and your household. And you shall not neglect the Levite who is within your towns, for he has no portion or inheritance with you.

God gave these people the option of paying their tithe by holding a celebration with family and neighbors in need. Explicitly mentioned among the things they might want to buy for their celebration are wine (*yayin* in Hebrew—the same *yayin* with which Noah sinned by becoming drunk in Genesis 9) and strong drink, also sometimes translated as "beer" (*shekar* in Hebrew, a fermented or distilled beverage made from grain, fruit, or honey).[1]

Psalm 104:15 speaks with praise of God's provision of "wine to gladden the heart of man, oil to make his face shine and bread to strengthen man's heart." Wine is also one of the elements on Lady Wisdom's table (Proverbs 9:2,5), and appears to have been a common beverage in Israelite society (1 Samuel 10:3; 16:20; 1 Chronicles 12:40; 27:27).

In the New Testament, Jesus apparently partook of wine throughout his time in the ministry, and was accused by his enemies of being a "glutton and a drunkard" for partaking instead of abstaining (Matthew 11:18-19). His first miracle in Cana was to turn water into wine in a celebratory environment—and not just wine [*oinos* in the Greek], but *good* wine (John 2:1-11). His last meal with the 12 disciples featured wine, with Jesus mentioning that he wouldn't drink it with them again until the great feast when the kingdom of God comes in all its fullness (Matthew 26:29; Mark 14:25).

The Bible condemns drunkenness.

Very compelling evidence for the idea that Christians are allowed moderate alcohol consumption are all the verses condemning drunkenness. The same word used in the Old Testament so positively in some verses of Proverbs, *yayin*, is also used with a warning in Proverbs 20:1: "Wine is a mocker, strong drink a brawler, and whoever is led astray by it is not wise." Isaiah speaks condemningly of people who "rise early in the morning, that they may run after strong drink [*shekar*], who tarry late into the evening as wine [*yayin*] inflames them!" (5:11). In Paul's letter to the Ephesians, he forbids readers to be drunk with "wine" (*oinos*) (5:18). This is the same substance that Jesus made out of water.

To me, the presence of these warnings is as compelling as the presence of positive-use descriptions of *yayin*, *shekar*, and *oinos*. These verses tell me, first, that we're talking about the same substances, and second, that our use of these substances has some very clear boundaries placed around them in Scripture.[2]

You can see that I am very much for the moderationist view of alcohol. I myself partake of it, and I have many Christian friends who do the same. This chapter is primarily written to the moderationist partaker. It is meant to offer some careful suggestions for godly practice and enjoyment of God's good gift. As Paul says, "For everything created by God is good, and nothing is to be rejected if it is received with thanksgiving, for it is made holy by the word of God and prayer" (1 Timothy 4:4-5).

But I also have a good many Christian friends who abstain, and I honor them. The Christian who abstains may have any number of good reasons for doing so. She may abstain on very good legal or health-related grounds, because she's underage, pregnant, or breastfeeding. Or perhaps she has a "weak conscience," such as Paul describes in Romans 14. She cannot partake of alcohol without a feeling that she has sinned because of some theological hang-up or association. She may have a weakness of self-control, and know it, and abstain for that reason. She knows that if she has one, she won't be able to stop. There may be a background of alcoholism in her family or in her own past, and she fears to replicate it.

She may also abstain because of the prevalence of drinking in our secular Western culture. She wants to be distinguished from the world, and alcohol abuse is so rampant that she doesn't feel up to the task of separating the alcohol from the abuse in her Christian witness. So, she abstains.

A Christian may also strategically abstain on specific occasions when she knows she'll be with brothers and sisters who are given to overdrinking or have captive consciences. This is my own practice (more on that in a minute). So, while freedom in moderation is my view here, and I think it lines up with Scripture, in my own practice I seek to reflect the nuance and love modeled in the same Word that gives me freedom to partake.

Pruning Fruitless Branches

In my backyard next to the chicken house, there are two fruit trees growing toward each other. Their trunks come out of the ground at a full 45-degree angle, about five feet apart. Their branches become entangled halfway up and are almost indistinguishable; this makes it the most romantic set of trees I've ever seen. They are literally combined at the hip. You can't tell where one tree ends and the other begins—the trees are married and grown in together.

I don't know what kind of fruit these trees will bear. The man who sold us the house gestured into the backyard loosely and mentioned the three fruit trees and said something about plums and something about apples, and I seem to remember something about peaches but am not too sure. Then the neighbors came by and mentioned the third tree standing nearby, identifying it as a plum tree that bears more plums than they've ever seen.

But the identity of the ingrown love trees is still a mystery. I wait for the spring when buds may tell me something, and I wait eagerly for the fall when something may appear that I can eat and feed to my fruit-loving girls. In the meantime, friends of mine who are serious gardeners have come over and pointed out how thick the branches are on the love trees; they need pruning.

So, naturally, last summer I googled "how to prune" and grabbed some shears and lugged my pregnant belly into the backyard. With a three-year-old and a two-year-old playing nearby, I clipped for hours. According to what I read, you get rid of branches that are clearly dead, branches that touch or entangle each other, and branches that can't get any light because they're inward facing. You want to have a clear path through your tree that a bird could conceivably fly through. Given a choice, you clip off branches that grow downward, and keep branches that grow upward toward the light.

I can't believe how hard it is to clip off branches that are clearly healthy, fine, live shoots. At first, I could hardly bring myself to do it. Never mind that the experts told me these branches are leaching energy from the tree. Never mind that I know if I fail to lop them off, energy will be diverted into the useless inner branches and away from the fruit I want. It's just hard. When I cut the branch, it feels like I'm cutting something off that is perfectly healthy and good and didn't do me any harm. It feels like killing, when it's actually promoting life.

The fruit tree's purpose is to make fruit. But if it stops making fruit, it's good for nothing but to be cut down and thrown into the fire. You must see where I'm going with this.

> "I am the true vine, and my Father is the vinedresser," says Jesus. "Every branch in me that does not bear fruit he takes away, and every branch that does bear fruit he prunes, that it may bear more fruit. Already you are clean because of the word that I have spoken to you. Abide in me, and I in you. As the branch cannot bear fruit by itself, unless it abides in the vine, neither can you, unless you abide in me. I am the vine; you are the branches. Whoever abides in me and I in him, he it is that bears much fruit, for apart from me you can do nothing" (John 15:1-5).

Fruit is what we were made to produce. Anything that stops us from bearing fruit needs to be cut off, even if it's otherwise a good-looking branch in our lives. But if we abide in him, we'll welcome this pruning. The pruning is proof of the fact that we're his, that we're under construction, that we're being cultivated. The pruning is a good thing.

I bring up the pruning not only because this is a vine reference and therefore a wine reference. I bring up pruning because I want to put us into a good position for recognizing if alcohol is a shoot in our lives that's growing the wrong way and needs to be cut off. If the branch of alcohol is strong and vibrant but growing funkily, low to the ground, trying to intertwine itself unhelpfully to the underside of another fruitful branch that's getting plenty of sunlight, it's possible that the alcohol branch needs to be lopped off. Maybe it's growing wrong.

You may feel like it's a step backward in your sanctification—*I'm supposed to be getting stronger, not weaker! I'm supposed to be able to handle things like this, things that God gave to be taken with thanksgiving! I'm supposed to be filled with the fruit of the spirit—self-control!*

But it's not a step backward in sanctification to pay attention to branches that need to be lopped off. They are fruitless. If they are fruitless, they are leaching good nutrients away from the places where fruit could be growing. They may grow back. And if so, they may grow back rightly—in position to grow straight and long and into the sunlight where they can bear fruit. But you aren't going to be able to move forward as a fruit tree when you give special exemptions to branches that are crookedly growing in the dark and need to be lopped off.

I'm a Christian woman who partakes of alcohol. I enjoy the celebratory atmosphere created in a group of friends enjoying good food and good drink together. I am married to a craft beer aficionado. I grew up in a Christian home where very temperate, even delicate, wine drinking was modeled by my mother (one glass, about twice a year).

But I am finding, along with a good friend of mine who has one of the most temperate, finely tuned palates around for alcohol I've seen, that "you just have to always keep watch." I've grown concerned during several seasons of my life that my private habits were creeping in the direction of dependency. And since I believe that I must not "be dominated by anything" (1 Corinthians 6:12), I keep a close watch on myself and discipline my body—belly and tongue too—lest I should be disqualified (1 Corinthians 9:27).

I've lopped off the branch of alcohol before for a season, and

I'm aware that I may have to do so again. I'm also standing at the ready, prepared to make a permanent cut for the sake of my spiritual state. Alcohol is a gift, but it's not a gift that can be allowed to interfere with the stated commands of the Giver. I have my marching orders. God has commanded me to walk temperately, to love sacrificially, to exercise self-control, and to live in a state of watchfulness for his coming. Drunkenness and watchfulness are not bedfellows. If alcohol is inhibiting me from fulfilling my marching orders, alcohol goes.

The Woman Wino Joke

I live in a small town in a dry county surrounded by dry counties. There's a privately owned pharmacy in the middle of a neighboring town where shoppers browse through southern chic home decor while their prescriptions are filled.

Between pillows and cake stands, two shelves are devoted to a tongue-in-cheek line of wine products. Wine glasses bear messages like "W.I.N.O.S.—Women In Need Of Sanity," "Hakuna Moscado: it means drink wine," and "Drink Like a Mother." Mugs and travel mugs are inscribed in cute fonts with "There's a good chance this is wine" and "COFFEE keeps me going until it is acceptable to drink WINE."

Online, Christian friends are sharing memes: "MOTHERHOOD: powered by love, fueled by coffee, sustained by wine."

I am a pastor's wife in a church where we have a healthy mixture of abstentionists and moderationists. It makes me very glad to see the ways that the drinkers and nondrinkers live and worship and work together in our midst. We have so many opportunities to practice love and grace with one another because of these kinds of differences—the kind that affect your dinner table on a Friday night.

I see it as our job to exhort one another and to set the example for one another about how to act and talk around alcohol in various settings. There are several levels that need to be addressed here: our private alcohol use, our use of alcohol around unbelievers, our use of alcohol around believers, and our habits of communication, both online and in person.

The woman wino joke described above is something to address first off because I think that this kind of talk often betrays a deeper problem. The ways we joke tend to betray the ways that we are struggling with sin. For, as we know, out of the abundance of the heart the mouth speaks (Luke 6:45). The woman wino joke communicates something rather painful—*life is hard, so hard that we might need alcohol to get through it*—in a way that relieves pressure, normalizes the feelings described, and allows us to sympathize with each other.

The jokes arise out of a gleeful love for the freedom we find to eat and drink, for "God has already approved what [we] do" (Ecclesiastes 9:7). But it's possible—just possible, that this kind of talk and the gleeful carelessness toward alcohol that may accompany it—is hurting our witness and hurting our brothers and sisters in Christ. So, let's ask God to "set a guard" over "the door of [our] lips" (Psalm 141:3), and submit our joking and our drinking to the Holy Spirit for inspection:

1. Do we drink and joke with love for our fellow drinking Christian women?

"I laugh at the jokes, but I don't appreciate them," said one mom, a Christian who confided that she was starting to wonder just this last winter if she was overdrinking. "They really aren't a good thing, although we laugh—because we're misleading each other. We're saying that we need wine in order to make it. We're saying that it's okay to use wine in order to make it."

The thing about any kind of joking that makes light of sin (in the case of some of these jokes, the sin of drunkenness) is that we are sending messages to each other about what God is capable of doing for us and what kind of behavior is seemly for the Christian. And these messages can be very unhelpful for someone who is struggling with sin.

"I started noticing recently that I wasn't just having a glass now and then. It was getting to be like every night of the week…and not just one glass but one, two, or three," said my friend. "And one day I was noticing that third glass and thinking, *This is probably not a good thing. I shouldn't need this.*"

The jokes about "mommy juice" are funny because we all get it—destressing is wonderful, and wine is stress relief in a bottle. The problem is that these jokes are a form of exhortation. What they communicate, essentially, is this: "The Holy Spirit is not sufficient for you. What you need is wine."

It's a missed opportunity, a pointing in the wrong direction, to be pretending with our sisters that anything can be sustained by wine. Wine, to the partaking Christian, is a gift to be accepted with thanksgiving. But it will not sustain us through the difficult days of relational trouble, deadlines, noise, and mess. God gave wine "to gladden the heart of man" (Psalm 104:15), but wine can never produce the joy that is brought by the Holy Spirit and that is stirred up as we gaze on Christ the Savior.

When we drink with our fellow women, or when we joke with our fellow women, we're responsible for the exhortations implicit in our behavior and our words. We're telling each other—in a million tiny ways—what our hope is. And if we lean into alcohol or coarse jokes about alcohol, we miss opportunities to exhort one another in ways that actually help.

We could be talking about how the love of Christ sustained us through a hard afternoon, how prayer was the lifeline that brought us through a terrible week, how obedience to discipline in love brought blessing that we didn't expect. Instead, we may be drinking or speaking in ways that could actually normalize alcohol abuse for a friend who is secretly struggling. And if we're overdrinking ourselves, then the joke isn't even the first sin that needs addressing. We're playing with fire that we've been warned about throughout Scripture. It doesn't need to be winked about; it needs to be killed (before it kills us).

2. Do we drink and joke with love for unbelievers?

Woman wino culture, with its attendant genre of jokes, is getting concerned secular attention right now.

"As a mother, I find that the number of demands put upon me in a single week is dizzying and never-ending," confessed Sarah Cottrell on *Babble*. "From financial stress to house stress to constantly feeling like I'm not the mother that I could or should be...the list of pressures and impending deadlines pile up. And so, like a lot of moms at the end of a long day, I turn to the internet and my nightly wine and seek comfort in knowing my problems also belong to others. Memes, blogs, all those snarky and witty women with clean houses and bold statements of being a 'hot mess' but 'have some wine' has become so normalized, I somehow didn't see it when my one glass of wine turned to five each night."[3]

Liz Tracy wrote about the issue in the *New York Times*, concluding that, as a nondrinker, she must look to other ways of fighting stress. "My vice is PBS murder mysteries," she said. "I also take antidepressants, do talk therapy, write and splurge on some indulgences at the grocery store."[4] To the believer who knows that Christ renews our minds, restores our souls, and strengthens us over time through a process called sanctification, these solutions might sound singularly ineffectual. But to the extent that we're willing to enter into the spirit of the wino meme, we are publicly offering a solution even less helpful than PBS murder mysteries and talk therapy.

Just as these jokes send a message to our believing friends, they send a message to our nonbelieving friends—not to mention strangers—online. The message is loud and clear: "Christ isn't going to help you. He hasn't helped us. Look! We still need wine to get through the everyday struggles of life." The way we drink and the way we speak about alcohol send a message, loud and clear, about what Christ has or hasn't done for us. And we have so much more to share.

3. Do we drink and joke with love for fellow Christians who abstain?

We've gone through many of the reasons that Christians have for abstaining from alcohol. And there are more we haven't mentioned, I'm sure. But the main thing we need to know is this: Our clearest instructions about eating and drinking in the New Testament have to do with our brothers and sisters. Paul's instructions for loving these people, whatever their personal or theological backgrounds, are as clear (and repeated) as almost anything he writes to his planted churches.

Our self-control at the table matters, and it is one palpable, physical way to demonstrate our love for one another. Paul has a warning for each of us who think that our brothers and sisters just need to "get over" their conscience hang-ups, and that this beer on the menu is just too good to wait while they do:

> The kingdom of God is not a matter of eating and drinking but of righteousness and peace and joy in the Holy Spirit. Whoever thus serves Christ is acceptable to God and approved by men. So then let us pursue what makes for peace and for mutual upbuilding. Do not, for the

sake of food, destroy the work of God. Everything is indeed clean, but it is wrong for anyone to make another stumble by what he eats. It is good not to eat meat or drink wine or do anything that causes your brother to stumble (Romans 14:17-21).

The spirit of this passage is clear: Our liberty always gives way to love. This means that while merlot is good, it's better for us to forego the merlot when we're sitting down to eat with someone who has a complicated history with alcohol. If you don't know someone's history or their stance on the issue, it's best to abstain rather than inadvertently causing them to stumble. While eating and drinking with thankfulness is good, that good is always second best to showing care and consideration for one another.[5]

Freedom in Christ

The glorious thing about our freedom is that it looks and sounds nothing like the world's freedom to get drunk and be the selves that have been bottled up in there waiting to be set free. "For freedom Christ has set us free...Only do not use your freedom as an opportunity for the flesh, but through love serve one another" (Galatians 5:1,13).

"Wine is how classy people get drunk" is the wisdom of the world (and overlooks the glaring question of whether "classy people," whatever that means, get drunk at all). Freedom, then, is not the selfish, reckless wielding of cravings and opinions. Freedom is the sober, calculated, sacrificial laying down of our lives for the good of others.

> Do not get drunk with wine, for that is debauchery, but be filled with the Spirit, addressing one another in psalms and hymns and spiritual songs, singing and

making melody to the Lord with your heart, giving
thanks always and for everything to God the Father in
the name of our Lord Jesus Christ, submitting to one
another out of reverence for Christ (Ephesians 5:18-21).

If that doesn't sound like freedom to us, then we may have had
a few too many glasses of what the world is serving.

We rejoice, whether it is in the pew or around the table. We
rejoice, whether over a glass of water or a glass of cabernet. We
rejoice, knowing our lives are not powered by coffee and sustained
by wine, but that they are powered and sustained by the oaths of
God. We have fled for refuge to Christ, and because of God's promises, we have strong encouragement to hold fast to the hope set
before us—a "sure and steadfast anchor of the soul," according to
Hebrews 6:19.

FOOD FOR THOUGHT

Discuss
- What is your current position on alcohol, and what are your personal practices?
- If you were dallying with the drunkenness condemned in Scripture, how would you know it? What is the line you currently draw for sin in this area?
- Would you be willing to cut alcohol out of your life if you found it was deterring you in your pursuit of Christ?
- If you are an abstainer, do you know Christians who are drinkers? How do you handle this area of differing practice?

Practice
- If you are an imbiber of alcohol, set up an occasion for imbibing with friends, using the occasion to watch your own habits and reflect on them. Have you been led to say anything you shouldn't? Have you been led to overdrink or overeat by the presence of alcohol? This is the moment to consider whether the wine has gladdened your heart as it was designed to, or deadened your awareness and made you a sitting duck for Satan's devices.

Read
- Read "Christians and Alcohol," an article by Tim Challies, for a helpful observation about generational differences on this issue and personal reflection on whether we youngish Christians should check our attitudes.[6]
- Watch two talks given by Joe Rigney for Bethlehem College, "On Alcohol" in two parts, for a balanced rundown of four possible positions on alcohol for the Christian—two of them legitimate, and two illegitimate.[7]
- Read *Addictions: A Banquet in the Grave*, Ed Welch's helpful biblical counseling manual on addiction.[8]

CHAPTER 9

Awakening Appetite

FASTING AS A SPIRITUAL PRACTICE

The real secret of fasting is not that it is a simple way to keep one's weight down, but that it is a mysterious way of lifting creation into the Supper of the Lamb.

—ROBERT F. CAPON, *THE SUPPER OF THE LAMB*[1]

From Memory: 2005

Day ten are the first words that form in my mind. My eyelids open instantly. My arms are weak as I drag the covers off of my legs and swing them to the side of the bed. I'm light-headed for just one second, and not from sleepiness—if anything, I'm unusually alert. I tiptoe carefully down the hallway and stairs and into the bathroom where the scale sits.

I'm 17, and I shamefully brought home 25 extra pounds at the end of my freshman year of college. This summer, I can think of nothing but those pounds. How to get them off? How? *How?* But according to the scale, this is how.

Those who care enough can always find a way, I think to myself.

In two long and hollow weeks on nothing but water, I will lose 20 of those pounds. I will feel certain that I've unlocked the secret.

I'll have spent all my time on the fast reading and watching TV and lounging around waiting for time to pass. Perhaps I should have prayed more, but I could think of nothing to pray about.

Why Should We Fast?

When could there ever be a time to abstain from a good gift God himself has given? The reasons for abstaining from food—the good reasons—are spiritual. They are reasons that have to do with turning from one kind of sustenance to another kind of sustenance. They have to do with pulling away from one kind of enjoyment in order to encounter a stronger, more lasting kind of enjoyment. They have to do with setting aside one good gift from God's hand in order to taste more fully of the Giver himself.

Fasting is also a way of reengaging the senses and reorienting the heart to thanksgiving. Most of our food problems, we've seen, are the problems of plenty rather than lack. We don't experience hunger from any circumstantial causes. Our lives, if we choose to live them this way, can easily be just one feast after another, ad nauseum. Exterior forces don't come along to deprive us of the steady stream of physical satisfaction; this means that if we ever want to experience hunger, we have to do it on purpose.

We know lots of reasons not to fast. Because it's hard, that's one reason. We also know from Scripture that there are bad reasons to fast, motives that should be actively avoided. We shouldn't fast to be seen by men, for instance. Jesus tells his followers that if they fast to be seen by men, they'll have all the reward (recognition) they're ever going to get and miss out on the true rewards of fasting, given by God himself (Matthew 6:16-18). We know that we're not to put God to the test (Luke 4:12)—so we can't fast to try to force God's hand on something.

With all these reasons not to fast, perhaps we need to spend our time here talking about reasons *to* fast. What could possibly tempt a Christian to voluntarily experience weakness, headaches, hunger pains, and deprivation? The enticements, come to find out, are great:

1. Fast to express our greater desire for God

This is the great reason to fast that changed my entire personal paradigm for fasting and was brought to my attention through John Piper's book *A Hunger for God*. This clarified for me—for the first time—what fasting is really all about.

Until last year (during a brief break between nursing and pregnancy), I'd been only vaguely familiar with the mechanics of fasting. I'd experienced a few vaguely purposed group fasts with fellow college ministry kids. But I never knew what you're supposed to *do* while you fast. How can it be a spiritual exercise when it's so very physical? The hunger was very real, but what else was I to expect?

I never understood how fasting could play a part of ordinary spiritual discipline in the Christian life, and how it could be associated most closely with *affection*. Piper's words about hunger for Christ awakened in me a desire to fast for reasons that were new to me:

> Fasting proves the presence, and fans the flame, of that hunger [for the supremacy of God]. It is an intensifier of spiritual desire. It is a faithful enemy of fatal bondage to innocent things. It is the physical exclamation point at the end of the sentence: "This much, O God, I long for you and for the manifestation of your glory in the world!"[2]

To have no other pressing reason for a fast—to fast simply as an expression of desire for God's presence and his glory—this was a new idea to me. I wanted new ways of waking up my affections for Christ when they felt dull. I wanted to have some spiritual practices that were a combination of spirit and body—acknowledgment that I have both a stomach and a heart, and that they both need to be brought under the lordship of Christ. This would be a new practice to me, and one I was so ready to toe into.

Piper's words encouraged me:

> The more deeply you walk with Christ, the hungrier you get for Christ...the more homesick you get for heaven...the more you want "all the fullness of God"...the more you want to be done with sin...the more you want the Bridegroom to come again...the more you want the Church revived and purified with the beauty of Jesus...the more you want a great awakening to God's reality in the cities...the more you want to see the light of the gospel of the glory of Christ penetrate the darkness of all the unreached peoples of the world...the more you want to see false worldviews yield to the force of Truth...the more you want to see pain relieved and tears wiped away and death destroyed...the more you long for every wrong to be made right and the justice and grace of God to fill the earth like the waters cover the sea.[3]

We get a subtle push from Jesus himself to fast, even in the same passage that warns against hypocritical fasting. "And *when you fast*," he says (notice the assumption that we, his followers, will at some point be fasting), "when you fast, do not look gloomy like the hypocrites, for they disfigure their faces that their fasting may be seen by others. Truly, I say to you, they have received their reward." What does this imply? It implies there's some other reward available, something they're missing: "But when you fast," he continues, "anoint your head and wash your face, that your fasting may not be seen by others but by your Father who is in secret. And your Father who sees in secret will reward you" (Matthew 6:16-18).

What's the reward? What can we expect from him when we fast? Why do we pass up this other reward (being seen and admired by men)? The reward is a reward to be found in the secret places. The reward is a reward of intimacy, a reward of knowing God himself better. There is a secret space we creep into with our fasting, a space for good desire to grow and lesser desire to weaken. His rewards there are rich and very personal. But they have nothing to do with points earned or reputation grown. They have to do with encountering the very face of God and expressing to him that he is our greatest need and desire.

Fasting is not just a way of expressing our desire for God. It's a way of stirring up that desire by suppressing the constant feeding of other (legitimate) needs. Food, you see, is essential to us. We're not going to make it very far without food; some superhuman efforts have resulted in just a few months or so. After three to five days of not eating, you may not feel so hungry, but you will start to feel a quiet sense of physical weakness that will remain with you until you break your fast.

Food is, under normal circumstances, actually essential to life. So, what fasting expresses and encourages is the sense that even though food is essential to us, God is more essential to us.

Man, you see, doesn't live on bread alone—but on every word that proceeds from the mouth of God (Matthew 4:4). And sometimes, our eager acceptance and enjoyment of innocent, good gifts from God stifles our acceptance and enjoyment of the richer table he lays out before us. The table of his Word is always available, but do we tuck into it with the same fervor that we tuck into our brownies and ice cream? Do we partake with the same sense of virtuous satisfaction with which we partake of our raw beans-and-greens salad and vegan dressing?

Sometimes, we lay aside God's good gifts to us (food, sex, entertainment, or even sleep) in order to taste and express hunger for Christ himself. In Piper's words, again:

> The greatest enemy of hunger for God is not poison but apple pie. It is not the banquet of the wicked that dulls our appetite for heaven, but endless nibbling at the table of the world. It is not the X-rated video, but the prime-time dribble of triviality we drink in every night. For all the ill that Satan can do, when God describes what keeps us from the banquet table of his love, it is a piece of land, a yoke of oxen, and a wife (Luke 14:18-20).[4]

Cornelius Plantinga Jr. echoed this idea:

> Self-indulgence is the enemy of gratitude, and self-discipline usually its friend and generator. That is why gluttony is a deadly sin. The early desert fathers believed that a person's appetites are linked: full stomachs and jaded palates take the edge from our hunger and thirst for righteousness. They spoil the appetite for God.[5]

We modern Western Christians may be good at a lot of things, but hunger is not one of them. Hunger for God—our greatest Good—will never grow if it is constantly stifled by lesser goods.

2. Fast to express sorrow

We see sorrowful fasting modeled often in Scripture: fasting to express sorrow over sin or over circumstances. David's most anguished fasting, as described in Scripture, occurred in sorrow over both sin and circumstances. Second Samuel tells the story of David taking Bathsheba from her husband and then compounding his first sin with murder. The prophet Nathan confronts David, and David admits his fault; then Nathan tells him that the son conceived with Bathsheba will die. When the son gets sick, David fasts in anguish for a week. The fast is an emotional and natural response to an emergency: David has sinned and is broken by his sin. David is experiencing loss, or the threat of loss, and is broken by that too (2 Samuel 11–12).

Fasting is a natural response to sin and to suffering. It is more natural in situations that are exceptional: a diagnosis, a death, a life-altering fall into sin or conviction of a long-term sin stronghold, a national emergency. Many of the corporate fasts called for in Scripture have to do with large-scale threats or decisions, such as when Esther calls her people to fast when they're threatened with genocide (Esther 4:15-16).

Likewise, our brokenhearted fasting could be either private or corporate. We could fast when we get bad news, or we could fast with our church to pray for the lives of the unborn millions being slaughtered every day. We could fast to express sorrow over conviction of sin, or we could fast to express sorrow over unrepentant sin in another. We could fast over natural disaster or human evil, our suffering or collective suffering.

In a sense, this is one of the clearest motives for fasting that Jesus presents when he's asked about fasting. John's disciples had come to him, asking why they and the Pharisees fasted regularly, but Jesus's own disciples didn't fast. And he said to them matter-of-factly, "Can the wedding guests mourn as long as the bridegroom is with them? The days will come when the bridegroom is taken away from them, and then they will fast" (Matthew 9:14-15).

In other words, *now is not the time*. It's as if Jesus is saying, "The time is coming. I'm here now, but I'm going to be going away again, and my people will be waiting for me. That's the time for fasting—that's the time for expressions of loss and longing, of groaning and readiness. My disciples don't fast while they're with me, but my disciples will certainly fast when they're wishing they were with me."

3. Fast to intensify prayer

Fasting and prayer are always associated in Scripture. We fast and we talk to God; the one without the other becomes meaningless ritual. It's impossible to talk about fasting without connecting it to prayer.

Even the last point, about fasting in sorrow, is difficult to distinguish from fasting in prayer—because after all, when we fast in sorrow, we are driven to ask God for intervention in the thing that has brought sorrow. If it's sin, we're driven to pray for repentance, forgiveness, restoration; if it's some other suffering, we're driven to ask for intervention, comfort, healing. Either way, the prayer and the fasting go hand in hand.

Fasting can be an expression of the intensity of our need in the thing we're praying for. But fasting can also be a way of ratcheting up our own sense of the need—of focusing our own hearts into lasers when they are more naturally strobe lights. Our thoughts are scattered and diffused everywhere—by tasks, people, desires, and shallow distractions. Sometimes we intend to pray for something, and it's a need we do care about—but we find when it comes right down to it that our "caring" about something is relative and transient. An urgent need in the church becomes less pressing than an urgent need to make a snack and sit down for a little e-mailing; the pressing desire we have to use today as a day of prayer for missions becomes a pressing desire to get to the laundry before the kids get home from school.

Sometimes our hearts need a little help to regain their sense of urgency in prayer. Fasting is a wonderful aid in this. Just as it intensifies and expresses our need to connect to the presence of Jesus himself, fasting intensifies and expresses our urgency in praying.

You may be distracted in fasting by weakness, headaches, or other physical effects of hunger, but one thing you won't do is forget that something different is happening today. Today, you are praying for the situation in Chad, or for your brother's marriage, or for revival in your congregation. Remember?

Many people use time they would have used on food to pray; this is helpful for the busy. It is also helpful even for those (like myself) who can't use time I would have used on food because I have a family to prepare food for. I can't stop making food. But I can certainly be taught by the fast to steal away extra moments and spend them on the business of the day.

If we're weak in prayer, perhaps a regular fast day would be a good way to grow in prayer over time. Our halfheartedness in praying may just be a symptom of our halfheartedness generally, and nothing wakes you up like hunger.

There's a story in 2 Kings about the prophet Elisha on his deathbed talking to King Joash of Israel. Joash is being faced with defeat by the armies of Syria. Elisha tells him to shoot an arrow out the window, and then tells him to take a handful of arrows and strike the ground with them. Joash strikes the ground three times and then stops. Elisha rebukes Joash: "You should have struck five or six times; then you would have struck down Syria until you had made an end of it, but now you will strike down Syria only three times" (2 Kings 13:14-20).

Perhaps this seems arbitrary, but Joash's halfhearted striking was a sign of a halfhearted request. He could have struck the ground with everything in him, begging like a person who cares. But he begged like a person who sort of cares. And apparently, this was offensive enough that God responded by giving him *sort of* a victory.

When we pray, we should be praying like people who care. And fasting can be an aid to us in that kind of prayer. Some of us are very good at "not my will but thine be done"—so good at it that we never engage in the kind of prayer that sweats blood.

4. Fast to show the body who's boss

This is a good opportunity to mention something that apparently crosses the mind of most women during discussions of fasting: *Fasting will help me lose weight!*

That summer during college when I lost a bunch of weight in two weeks on nothing but water, I was convinced I'd found the secret. But not only was there no spiritual benefit in that fast, there was no lasting weight loss either. The weight was back on with a vengeance by the time the fall semester began.

When I was converted several years later and spent several years working through my bulimia, I didn't try fasting again for some time. It was too dangerous. Fasting was impossible for me to disentangle from crash diets and from thoughts of taking off a few pounds quickly—I couldn't even imagine what it would be like to fast without bodily effects being the foremost thing in my mind.

Apparently, I'm not alone. Several adult women confessed this to me during a season when fasting was being taught at our church. Fasting and dieting are very difficult to separate, and they've been dieting for so long. How to set fasting apart? How can they make it a spiritual exercise when their minds and hearts have been trained to think in terms of weight loss for their entire adult lives?

Is there any reason to think of fasting as a physical training, similar to the way we think of diet and exercise? Is there any physical effect that we can accept as among the legitimate benefits of fasting?

My answer to this is very tentative, but based on my best understanding of Scripture, as well as personal experience.

In 1 Corinthians 9:25-27, Paul says:

> Every athlete exercises self-control in all things. They do it to receive a perishable wreath, but we an imperishable. So I do not run aimlessly; I do not box as one beating the air. But I discipline my body and keep it under control, lest after preaching to others I myself should be disqualified.

Notice that he specifically talks about disciplining his body here. He seems to believe that his body is given to wandering into sin and indulgence and needs to be kept "under control." And we know from experience that our bodies are this way—they have appetites, and those appetites are not given to easy governance. What our bodies often want in the way of sexual fulfillment, food, leisure, or entertainment is not always best. Sometimes, we have to tell our bodies what is best: the best time and context for sexual fulfillment, the best food for true enjoyment and sustenance, the best amount of work and leisure, and the best quantity and quality of entertainment. Our bodies don't always choose these things on their own.

But Paul, if you notice, is not primarily concerned with physical discipline leading to physical ends (athletic ones). He is concerned with physical discipline leading to spiritual ends: his ability to finish his race well, completing the good works that were ordained for him. So he wants to be able to do his job. This spiritual end (faithfulness in kingdom work) must be served at times by physical means (disciplining his body).

"An old saint once said that fasting prevents luxuries from becoming necessities," writes Jerry Falwell. "Fasting is a protection of the spirit against the encroachments of the body. When a person fasts, he has his body well in hand, and is able to do the work of the Master."[6] That's the thing I want you to remember when you're asking whether fasting is just another word for a really intense diet. In my experience, a fast can be entered into with vastly different aims, and you can come out the other end with vastly different effects. But just so you know, any weight loss from fasting—if you're given to overeating anyway and have been training yourself in a continual cycle of dieting and overdoing—is almost guaranteed to be temporary. Fasting is simply not a great way to approach weight loss.

But if you have goals of developing self-control—a spiritual end—through spiritual and physical means, then fasting may be one great way to approach that. Part of self-control is knowing what it feels like to tell our bodies *no* when we are used to telling them *yes*.

And there's no other way of strengthening such a skill but with practice. So if you want to think of fasting as one prong in the endeavor mentioned here by Paul—disciplining your body and keeping it under control, lest after preaching to others you yourself should be disqualified—that seems to me to be both legitimate and potentially helpful.

Remember though, that fasting is exactly like other spiritual disciplines: They are a means God uses to change you and help you know him better. But they are not a way you can bypass your relational problem with God (you don't love him enough) by going through physical motions (like giving, praying, or fasting).

Jesus warns us of this regularly in the Gospels. Remember the Pharisee: "God, I thank you that I am not like other men, extortioners, unjust, adulterers, or even like this tax collector. I fast twice a week; I give tithes of all that I get" (Luke 18:11-12). Apparently, it's quite possible to give and fast regularly without benefiting spiritually. The Pharisee managed it.

John Piper puts in his own warning about the dangers of spiritual pride in fasting:

> In the heart of the saint both eating and fasting are worship. Both magnify Christ. Both send the heart—grateful and yearning—to the Giver. Each has its appointed place, and each has its danger. The danger of eating is that we fall in love with the gift; the danger of fasting is that we belittle the gift and glory in our willpower.[7]

Just as it's possible to eat to the glory of God and fast to the glory of God, it's possible to fall into sin while doing either. Only our desire for intimacy with Christ can preserve us from feasting in idolatry or fasting in pride.

So, do you have a plan for fasting? Is it part of your life? The plan doesn't have to be ambitious, but perhaps a plan would bring fasting into your life as a spiritual practice for the long haul. This could help guard against a mind-set that believes *this fast, this week*, is going to solve all my dieting and self-control problems forever and get me into the body of my dreams.

5. Fast to prepare for obedience

The most terrifying passage about fasting in the Bible might be Isaiah 58. Read it to see what I mean:

> Cry aloud; do not hold back;
>   lift up your voice like a trumpet;
> declare to my people their transgression,
>   to the house of Jacob their sins.
> Yet they seek me daily
>   and delight to know my ways,
> as if they were a nation that did righteousness
>   and did not forsake the judgment of their God;

they ask of me righteous judgments;
  they delight to draw near to God.
"Why have we fasted, and you see it not?
  Why have we humbled ourselves, and you take no
    knowledge of it?"
Behold, in the day of your fast you seek your own pleasure,
  and oppress all your workers.
Behold, you fast only to quarrel and to fight
  and to hit with a wicked fist.
Fasting like yours this day
  will not make your voice to be heard on high.
Is such the fast that I choose,
  a day for a person to humble himself?
Is it to bow down his head like a reed,
  and to spread sackcloth and ashes under him?
Will you call this a fast,
  and a day acceptable to the LORD? (verses 1-5).

This first half of the passage is terrifying because it describes activities and postures that sound absolutely righteous and good to us. These are people who seek God daily and delight to know his ways? They are fasting and humbling themselves, and God is not hearing them? How is it possible?

In the passage, God calls the prophet to cry aloud what their transgression is. "This is why I don't hear you," he answers them. To paraphrase, he says, "I don't hear because even though you fast, you are still seeking your own pleasure, oppressing your workers, quarrelling and fighting, and hitting with a wicked fist."

Sarcastically, he asks if they think it's pleasing to him for them to be bowing and scraping like a reed, wearing sackcloth but undergoing no true repentance from their sins of oppression and self-service. And just when you start wondering—*What? What is it that they should do? What does he want; what would make their fasting a true fast?* He answers the question:

> Is not this the fast that I choose:
>   to loose the bonds of wickedness,
>   to undo the straps of the yoke,
> to let the oppressed go free,
>   and to break every yoke?
> Is it not to share your bread with the hungry
>   and bring the homeless poor into your house;
> when you see the naked, to cover him,
>   and not to hide yourself from your own flesh? (verses 6-7).

It seems from this passage that the biggest problem with their fasting is that they're insensitive to the needs of those in their care, and to those suffering whom they have the power to help. They fast, they seek holy habits, they study—but they don't care about bonds of wickedness, about oppressed people under a yoke. In their inaction, they are actively oppressing. In their selfishness with bread (even while fasting!), they ignore the hungry and homeless poor. They hide themselves from people who share the same flesh and blood. God urges them to hide their faces no longer, but to seek out the needs of others and fill them. A fast that is content to ignore these needs is no fast at all.

I've heard of Christians in developing countries fasting as a means of being generous. Living in places where their grain is allotted for exactly that day or that week, they are freer to share if they spend a day not eating. They take the rice they would have eaten that particular day and give it to neighbors in need. The fasting and the generosity are connected—so connected that the one makes the other possible.

If we see no connection between fasting and stoking the fires of generosity in our hearts and habits, we have misunderstood the nature of fasting. And moreover, we miss out on the blessings promised in the next verses of this chapter:

> Then shall your light break forth like the dawn,
>   and your healing shall spring up speedily;
> your righteousness shall go before you;
>   the glory of the LORD shall be your rear guard.
> Then you shall call, and the LORD will answer;
>   you shall cry, and he will say, "Here I am."
> If you take away the yoke from your midst,
>   the pointing of the finger, and speaking wickedness,
> if you pour yourself out for the hungry
>   and satisfy the desire of the afflicted,
> then shall your light rise in the darkness
>   and your gloom be as the noonday.
> And the LORD will guide you continually
>   and satisfy your desire in scorched places
> and make your bones strong;
>   and you shall be like a watered garden,
> like a spring of water,
>   whose waters do not fail (verses 8-11).

Perhaps, when you are praying for the needy during a fast, you could use some of your time asking for guidance in what needs to meet. We live in a globalized age. As Western Christians, our reach is almost unlimited; we can feed people in our neighborhoods, but we can also feasibly feed people across the world with clicks of a button. For many of us, there is a sense of helplessness in the face of so many options for generosity, and a sense of guilt because we know we're not doing what we could.

Fasting is a good time to focus in on this feeling, to lean into it in prayer and ask God what he would have us do. He does not intend for us to live with low-grade guilt, and there's nothing we can do to pay our way to a state of righteousness—in our backyards or across the globe. But if we have a guilty feeling that we are not generous enough with our time and resources, the guilty feeling may be present because we are actually guilty. Perhaps Isaiah 58 describes us perfectly—bowing our heads like reeds while hiding our faces from needs that are right in front of us.

Fasting can be an aid to action, or it can be a substitute for seeking God's preferred fast.

6. *Fast to reawaken appetite and thanksgiving*

There's no question about it: when you break a fast, you feel differently about food than you did before the fast. Your senses are reengaged and snapped out of boredom. Your heart is primed—if you've used the fast well, it's reoriented to thanksgiving.

Father Robert Capon has lots to say about fasting in *The Supper of the Lamb*; most of it had to do with fasting so that you can taste food better and fasting so that you are free to enjoy your food instead of eating pathetic diet stuff. Much of his advice skates a little too close, for me, to advice about how to "lose a few pounds without really trying." But I love what he has to say about reawakened appetite:

> I offer it as my prescription for Harry. Let him fast until he is free to eat like a true son of Adam. Let him take but one meal a day (or even one every other day, if he is one of the chosen ones whose metabolism marks him for a special vocation); let him fast in good earnest; nothing but liquids—no nibbles, no snacks. But then let him take meals worthy of the name...it is bread that strengthens man's heart; it is the valleys thick with grain that laugh and sing. It is only when Harry, by feast and fast,

lays a firm grip on the fatness of the earth, that he himself will return to sanity and substance.[8]

I've already said that Westerners don't do hunger well. One implication of this is that we can't possibly enjoy our food at maximum capacity. We are so used to abundance. An exercise in intentional hunger could help us to regain our enjoyment and retune our hearts to thanksgiving. How can we regain taste when tastelessness reigns? Capon continues:

> The real secret of fasting is not that it is a simple way to keep one's weight down, but that it is a mysterious way of lifting creation into the Supper of the Lamb. It is not a little excursion into the fashionable shape, but a major entrance into the fasting, the agony, the passion by which the Incarnate Word restores all things to the goodness God finds in them. It's as much an act of prayer as prayer itself, and, in an affluent society, it may well be the most meaningful of all the practices of religion—the most likely point at which the salt can find its savor once again. Let Harry fast in earnest, therefore. One way or another—here or hereafter—it will give him back his feasts.[9]

Fasting is not a way for us to forget the fact that, in the end of time, it's a feast we're waiting for. Fasting is actually a way to strengthen our readiness for that feast. Fasting is a way to get us hungry for food again, yes, but it's also a way to get us hungry for the real feast that's coming:

- A wedding feast prepared by a king, for which he has slaughtered oxen and fat calves and sent out invitations (Matthew 22:1-14).

- A banqueting house owned by our Lover and

Bridegroom, at which the decorations, the banner over our heads, will be love itself (Song of Solomon 2:4).

- A mountain feast laid by the LORD of hosts for all peoples, a feast of rich food, well-aged wine; a celebration of the new age where death is defeated finally; a feast where the people say, "Behold, this is our God; we have waited for him, that he might save us. This is the LORD; we have waited for him; let us be glad and rejoice in his salvation" (Isaiah 25:6-9).

In the end, the state we look forward to is not a state of fasting, but a state of feasting. We fast only in the absence of our Bridegroom, and we fast with the knowledge that someday we'll be glutted on his presence.

FOOD FOR THOUGHT

Discuss

- What has been your personal experience with fasting?

- What are some reasons for fasting that most intrigued you from this chapter?

- Why do you think many Christians don't practice fasting?

Practice

- Designate a time every month or every season for fasting. Start slow, with perhaps a one-day fast or a fast that is broken at suppertime.

- Use your fasts as opportunities for memorizing Scripture, interceding on behalf of someone you know, or pleading with God over something that is troubling you. Or spend your fasting time meditating on God in his Word or in a rich devotional book.

- Look up the World Vision and Feeding America websites for information on hunger relief overseas and at home.[10] Also look at Give Directly, an organization that sends cash directly to the world's poorest.[11] Prayerfully consider where your own resources of money and time should be spent.

Read

- Read *A Hunger for God* by John Piper, and perhaps plan to read this during your next fast. If you're not fasting while reading this book, it'll make you wish you were.

CHAPTER 10

Will Travel, Have Food

INTERNATIONAL CUISINE AND HEAVEN

The beer was very cold and wonderful to drink. The *pommes a l'huile* were firm and marinated and the olive oil delicious. I ground black pepper over the potatoes and moistened the bread in the olive oil. After the first heavy draft of beer I drank and ate very slowly.

—EARNEST HEMINGWAY, *A MOVEABLE FEAST*[1]

From Memory: 2008

I am standing in the cool air on cobblestones. Stone buildings stretch around the piazza, and none of them are buildings I've seen in a postcard or in a guide to Italian travel.

The men in Ascoli Piceno are striking. It takes me a while to understand what is so different about them, but then I realize: They dress so very well. The women are well dressed too, but women always take care of themselves. Here the men—old, young, rich, poor—they wear leather jackets and good dark-wash jeans, or good wool sweaters and well-made hats, and all of them with the best shoes and sunglasses. They are all handsome when young, and all very wrinkled in middle age, but still handsome.

I am standing in the square, embarrassed because I've just

noticed how hideous my black imitation Crocs are, and because I've just been overcome to the point of pulling out my camera and taking a picture, thus giving myself away officially as a tourist in a tourist-free zone. My hosts, parents of the children I'm temporarily nannying, are nearby buying these fried green olives that sound disgusting but turn out to taste more blissful and Italian than anything I've yet had. They have Parmigiano around them or inside of them and they are fried in oil and they collapse in your mouth.

A very handsome young Italian has been standing nearby, talking to another young Italian, but I have my back turned and am paying attention to the olives and the cobblestoned square. It is the second "Excuse me" before I notice the English and turn around. He looks into my eyes and holds eye contact, and he knows he's being charming like he's seen in a movie.

"Excuse me—where are you from?"

"America," I say.

"Oh," he says. He nods, holds my gaze, smiles again. "The olives," he gestures, "are very good."

I have to ask him to repeat this, and when I finally understand, I can only nod and say, "Yes—I mean si," and then he has nothing more to say. He tries a few lines from the Italian-to-English phrasebook, and we are at an impasse. I turn back to the olives and leave him and his friend standing in the square.

Keeping the Romance Alive

When I was 20 years old, I went to live in Italy for three months. I took a position as an au pair with a British family in a mountain village called Force. This is located in the Le Marche region of the country, which roughly approximates the middle calf of the boot, and which means I was a good several hours from any landmark city. (Rome is over on the shin of the boot, Venice is up on the back of the knee, Florence is landlocked above the calf, and Milan edges up into the thigh.) In other words, I wasn't going to see any other Americans for a long time.

I took care of two boys, ages five and three. The five-year-old, Lolli, was blind and autistic and a lover of the Bobs—Bob Dylan and Bob Marley. Arthur was the three-year-old, blonde, personable, and a royal terror most of the time. Their parents, I discovered after I arrived, were not married. They lived in silent British relational tension, supported by government money from two different countries due to Lolli's condition.

Force had about two cafés, a post office, a bakery, a produce shop, a school, a florist, and a few other shops. Just a few streets, sitting on top of a mountain, oriented around a large, lone Catholic church. The lifestyle was very provincial, which I enjoyed. We hung our washing outside or in front of the fire, we did dishes by hand, and we lit the stove with a match. When I made eggs in the morning, they were these rich-yolked, brown beauties from the chickens behind the house.

The bottom floor of our skinny, three-story house was a dungeon. To get to it, you had to climb down very steep stone steps into a room that looked like it must have been used to torture someone at some point. This was the kitchen and still something of a torture chamber because it was here that we ate our meals together.

Meals generally happened the same way. They began with a little period of quiet.

"Mmm...very good, Lolli," said my host mother, Monica. "Eat your porridge."

"I've got to go into town today; I'm doing a chair for Luca," from Harry.

It was about this time that Artie would decide to contribute to the conversation. He'd begin by looking directly at us, smiling sweetly, then screaming "Bloody hewl!" or "Fahty sh—!" or something similar. Monica and Harry would pretend not to hear him and speak very sweetly until Lolli joined in the noisemaking and Artie switched over to just a steady, incessant yell. Then one of the parents, usually Monica, would swing to the only possible extreme and yell, "Artie, *shut up*! You're *always* misbehaving, Artie, I don't understand why you must be *so naughty* all the time!"

It would go on this way for the rest of the meal. High, low, high, low; very loud, absurdly lenient; sweet and interesting, obnoxious and intentionally *cattivo* (naughty)...all of them in their own way. My heart would hurt for the boys at these mealtimes as I crunched my way through Monica's vegetarian, British-Italian cooking.

I was initially fascinated with the Britishness of my hosts, while also soaking up the sensations of the Italian countryside on my days off. The fact was, it was a terribly romantic place, and I'm sure this romance could have been preserved if it weren't for the people. But I began to realize soon after I came that these people I lived with were just like people at home (except when potty training they said things like "wee" and "willy" and "water closet"). I heartily wished for more teatime politeness and less ordinary squabbling. Instead, I discovered that one of the strange smells in the house was a result of my hosts' penchant for hand-rolled marijuana.

The Best Food I'll Never Eat Again

So I went looking for romance elsewhere. On the weekends and during a three-week stint at the end of my au pair engagement, I took trains to Florence, Venice, Milan, and Paris.

In Venice, I met an old man painting near the Plaza del Marco. We talked for an hour, and he showed me everything he had for sale—his work was entirely in sharp charcoal, very different from the oil paintings for sale everywhere up and down the canal. Beautiful. I wanted to see everything he had with him. He invited me to sit for a portrait the next day.

We met at noon and he brought me to Caffè Florian to meet friends and bought me a tiny little cup of dark coffee, which is the way the Italians do it. I spilled a little on the white tablecloth while showing him the pastels I'd been working on. He told me about famous people who had come to his booth on Piazza San Marco and bought his work—Robert Downey Jr. and other people who were famous in the 1990s. Then he led me through watery streets to a tiny garret where he proceeded to make clear that his usual way to paint models was in the nude. I declined, and he amicably did a clothed charcoal portrait. I loved his scenes of Venice, rendered in deft charcoal strokes, and I used up precious hostel money buying one of his pieces. He gave me another one to match, and the two pictures are in my dining room to this day. He was a lonely man and a massive Beatles fan. I was thankful that he was old because I would never have gone to his studio if he'd been young; even though he was a tad lascivious, I never felt like I was in danger at all.

In Milan, I had hosts for my first Christmas away from home. We ate very good food there, cooked by the matron of the house. She made spaghetti carbonara and did something with chicken that I have never seen since. When I arrived at their house, I brought a traditional cake-in-a-box because it was for sale in every train and bus station between Force and Milano. Panettone was piled everywhere you looked that Christmas—a light, naked, rounded cake with dried fruit in it, packed into individual cardboard boxes. Sometimes I see them in Aldi now. I don't know if that cake was any good, but I gave a few of my precious food euros for it so I wouldn't show up at their house empty-handed.

I rang in the new year in Paris in an apartment near the tenth arrondissement with a group of international Christian students.

In Paris, I didn't eat anything French or expensive because I had no money left. For two of the days I fasted on purpose because I had grown very fat in Force and was worried about the day I would go home. Other days, I bought a loaf of really disgusting German grain bread that was compact so I could carry it around the city with me, and some cheese and fruit. Every day I went out in the city and looked for where the romantic part of the city was—the warm part that had balconies with hanging baskets and sunsets over rooftops. I looked in the famous Shakespeare & Co. bookshop and on the lawn near the Eiffel Tower; I walked along the Seine looking for it. I climbed up into Montmartre, which overlooks the city, and I found some of it there. But on the whole, Paris was too cold to be romantic in January, and I was longing for home. Also, I made the mistake of buying a little Eiffel Tower keychain piece, and keychains have a way of removing any residual romance from your memory of a place.

In Florence, I had the one culinary experience that can never be recovered or repeated. At this time, my very favorite food in the world was ice cream. I was not embarrassed to say this to anyone. And I knew, before going to Italy, that Italian gelato was supposed to be the quintessential experience of ice cream as a food category. Well, just before I went to Florence, I heard that Italians considered Florentine gelato to be the best gelato, and moreover, there was a place in Florence that was considered by Florentines to be the best in the city. I don't remember the name of this shop now. Nor can I remember where it was in the city, and I imagine that in ten years, the gelato landscape has changed. But here's what I do know: I went into this shop and ordered a scoop of mint chip and a scoop of apple. And it was a perfect bowl, one flavor eaten to the end and then the other. I knew as I was eating that it was a pinnacle food experience. I was eating the best rendition in the best location of the best traditional form of my favorite food. And it was after a long, hard walk.

The Disappointment of Travel

We sent my mother to Paris a few years ago. All of her kids (she has seven of them) pooled their money together and bought a ticket for her to go with a friend. I wanted her to go for several reasons. She'd been a serious Francophile for as long as I could remember and has real French blood running in her veins, courtesy of the Baton Rouge Gremillion family. But with increased frequency the year we sent her, she'd been talking about Paris specifically. It was like she couldn't get it off her mind.

So I wanted her to go because she'd always wanted to go. But I also wanted her to find out the thing I'd learned by going to the places in my dreams—something I wasn't sure could be communicated any other way: You have to go to the place of your dreams to find out that heaven isn't located there.

When my mother went to Paris, she came back with a very similar attitude about Parisian jam that I have to Florentine gelato. She maintained that the jam in Paris was the best jam, and that there was no way to re-create the taste of the jam, even after she found and bought some of the same brands of jam as those she was eating in the Parisian cafés. And I believe her. There is something about food in a foreign place that becomes inimitable forever after. We know, after we've had the mountaintop experience of Pad Thai in that tiny place across the world, that no one can ever give this to us again. We will insist to our friends for the rest of our lives that nobody can make [blank] like the [blank] do. And logical statements about combining the same ingredients in the same way to the same effect won't budge us.

My mother is right. There's no jam like Parisian jam. There are no olives like those olives in Ascoli Piceno. There's no gelato like that gelato in Florence.

But you find out another important thing when you go to Paris.

You find out that whatever else the place is, it is not the place where all dreams come true and where your tears are wiped away. The longing that brings you to Paris still comes home with you. And it never leaves you. Not all the Parisian jam in the world can cure the hunger of your heart.

God and the Romance of Foreign Cuisine

What these travels can show us, first, is something about God himself. He loves variety, clearly, and he's capable of producing it in quantities beyond our wildest imaginations. He's the one who managed not only to make us and the cultures that incubated us, but the cultures that incubated a wider variety of communities and individuals than we're capable of imagining. He is responsible for the distinct cultures of the Incan Americans, the Bangkok Thai, the midcentury Parisian artists. Just as he found it worthwhile to extend his creative finger into the development of cinnamon, bay leaf, and saffron, he found it worthwhile to extend his creative finger into the development of the Samurai code of honor, the creek-bathing laundry day in India, the traditional pub full of old men in rural Ireland. The wealth of God's imagination created combinations of people and places and traditions that fill us with a combination of joy and longing.

But these travels also show us something about our appetite for God. Due to years of C.S. Lewis reading, I can never help but connect my attraction to foreign lands with my longing for God. In classic works like *Mere Christianity* and *The Weight of Glory*, Lewis argues from universal experience. He describes the human response of joy and hope that a foreign land stirs up in us, often from afar. We see a movie or read a book or see a photo, and from then on, we have a sketch in our minds about what a place feels like. It is, to us, Jane Austen's London. It is Jack London's or Anne of Green Gables's

Canada. It is the China of missionary Gladys Aylward. We long for the place, assuming that when we get there, the place will give us more of whatever we caught a glimpse of in that book or movie or photo. And when we get there, it just might. We may have the gelato to end every gelato. We may go on a gondola ride with a handsome stranger we'll never forget.

But if we hang around long enough, we'll see the place that actually exists beneath the romance. We'll hear the stranger talk about his mother and hear his funny cough. We'll get a job and have to go to work every day, and we'll stop noticing the watery streets. The place in our dreams will become another place where people are rude and where you have to drink coffee in order to get through the morning.

Lewis says that these experiences awaken hope in us—a hope that isn't ever quite consummated with a fulfillment of what is promised. He says this is evidence of our longing for God himself. "If I find in myself desires which nothing in this world can satisfy, the only logical explanation is that I was made for another world," he famously points out.[2]

This may seem like pixie-tailed, wishful thinking. But, as Lewis counters, our having stomachs means at the very least that food exists somewhere, and that stomachs were made to be fed. We may starve to death—people sometimes do—but our stomachs will protest about it because stomachs know what they were made for. We hunger, and our hunger is evidence not just of the fact that we have stomachs, but of the fact that there is something called food.

In the end, our search for transcendent joy is an indicator that we have souls. That's as simple as it gets. We may not get a happy ending to our stories, but the fact that people watch romantic comedies set in New York City says we were designed for a happy ending. We were designed to pursue joy, with the same concentration of purpose with which our stomachs pursue food.

And sometimes, we pursue joy *in* our food. But just as food will let us down, the romance of a food destination will let us down.

To the extent that we know a place, to that exact extent do we discover the brokenness of the people in that place. The more familiar it becomes to us, the more its honeymoon sheen wears off, and we discover that it's just exactly like home but with different vowel sounds. People are people, and people are a joy. But people are also a pain, a drain. Even if we didn't find this to be true of people we encountered in a new place, we'd still have to deal with the fact that we ourselves had followed ourselves here. And our own hearts bring enough of the nastiness to embitter our experience.

We always find that a place we were assured was heaven is not in fact heaven at all. And heaven, to be perfectly clear, is what we require. It's the beauty that we desire, but it's also the element of newness, the one that continually slips away with time. We can find beauty in our own town, but we can't find that sense of transportation or transformation. We want the Other of a place that is totally unlike the one we live in now.

When we pursue travel with such intensity, it's not because we love planes, trains, and automobiles. It's because of heaven. We hope that these places will answer the spiritual homelessness. Perhaps these places will reveal to us the secret meaning and pleasure that all along we've felt ourselves to be born for. We experience food in places like these and stuff those culinary experiences with the hope of salvation. The food is emblematic of the place that we're trying to believe is heaven. We tell stories of the secret pasta in the secret family-owned hole-in-the-wall, the suckling pig that was smoked for three days on an island beach. They are a measurement of the success of our travels; they're a token of our pilgrimage. They are evidence of the heaven we almost found.

But we do wonder—when will that heaven come? Where is the place we'll sit and eat our fill, the land of beauty that doesn't fade? When will we be surrounded by people who don't get uglier on acquaintance, people whose natures are supplied by some other substance than dirt, people who make up some long-lost community of love, joy, peace, patience, kindness, goodness, faithfulness, gentleness, and self-control? And where is the locus of the longing—the Being who is supposed to be waiting for us at the banquet table in our dreams?

"If you knew where the good water was to be found, you wouldn't waste your time pursuing this well water," says Jesus to the Samaritan woman (in so many words). He adds, "Whoever drinks of the water that I will give him will never be thirsty again. The water that I will give him will become in him a spring of water welling up to eternal life" (John 4:14).

"Blessed is everyone who will eat bread in the kingdom of God!" (Luke 14:15) exclaims a disciple, reclining at the table with the one whose body will soon be bread.

"My soul will be satisfied as with fat and rich food, and my mouth will praise you with joyful lips," says the psalmist (Psalm 63:5).

"Come, everyone who thirsts, come to the waters; and he who has no money, come, buy and eat!" says the prophet. "Come, buy wine and milk without money and without price. Why do you spend your money for that which is not bread, and your labor for that which does not satisfy? Listen diligently to me, and eat what is good, and delight yourselves in rich food" (Isaiah 55:1-2).

We wait to be satisfied with rich food, to eat bread in the kingdom of heaven. We long to drink fully of that water that will stop us being thirsty ever again. We sit down and taste, and our appetites grow larger even as they are sated. Rome hasn't satisfied us. Paris hasn't been the abundance we searched for. Our home, we see now, is elsewhere. Our table, we understand, is laid and waiting for us in another place.

Discuss

- Name a place you've always dreamed of going. What are the specific images you have of that place that attract you?

- See if you can connect heaven to that earthly place you have always wanted to go. Is there something (or someone) you hope to find in heaven that will answer that call in your heart?

Practice

- Look up the recipe online for "Ascoli fried olives." Apparently, those olives I had in the square have become famous across Italy, but it looks like you need about 12 hours and chef's training to make them.

- Book a flight, if you like (and bring me back some olives). Just don't forget where heaven isn't.

Read

- Enjoy *A Moveable Feast* by Ernest Hemingway for a sensory description of Paris during the 1920s.

- Dive into *Mere Christianity* by C.S. Lewis, for more on this connection between travel and heaven.

CHAPTER 11

Taste and See

THE LORD'S TABLE

When he had given thanks, he broke it, and said, "This is my body, which is for you. Do this in remembrance of me."

—1 CORINTHIANS 11:24

From Memory: April 2018

I'm sitting on a lawn chair in the front yard. My three-year-old plays in the dirt nearby. She straightens from a crouching position and comes toward me, holding a thimble-sized cup made of an acorn.

"Here, Mommy," she says. "Drink it. It's fox blood."

A shudder goes through me at the abrupt introduction of violence into a beautiful spring day.

"Fox blood?" I say, snorting. "Why is it fox blood? We don't drink blood, honey."

"Yes, we do," she patiently tells me. "We drink Jesus's blood at church. See? So it's fox blood; you can drink it."

"Oh," I say.

The Violent Feast to End All Violence

The followers of Jesus experienced a similar reaction to similar language in John 6. After Jesus broke bread to feed thousands on a hillside, the people became very enthusiastic about him. They would have taken him by force to make him their king if he hadn't slipped away.

But the next day, the crowd found him again, pursuing him in boats. He gave them a little shake-of-the-head kind of speech: "Truly, truly, I say to you, you are seeking me, not because you saw signs, but because you ate your fill of the loaves. Do not labor for the food that perishes, but for the food that endures to eternal life, which the Son of Man will give to you. For on him God the Father has set his seal" (John 6:26-27).

So they asked him what they should do, then, and he answered that the work of God was to believe in the one God sent. Yes, they said, *That's nice, but God used to feed his people bread in the wilderness—manna, remember that?—so hey, we wouldn't mind if you got in on the manna business too.* He'd already given them some excellent miracle barley bread at this point, so you can see why they were still a little distracted. *Try and focus,* he said to them, in effect. "It was not Moses who gave you the bread from heaven, but my Father gives you the true bread from heaven" (John 6:32).

"Sir, give us this bread always," they responded immediately. And this is where he really opened things up to them. He told them that he was the bread of life, and anyone who came to him would no longer hunger or thirst. He talked to them some more about God having sent him, and that his job was to keep and raise to life those God gave him. He talked about how nobody could come unless they were drawn, and then he returned again to this language about belief and eating:

> "I am the bread of life," he said again. "Your fathers ate the manna in the wilderness, and they died. This is the

bread that comes down from heaven, so that one may eat of it and not die. I am the living bread that came down from heaven. If anyone eats of this bread, he will live forever. And the bread that I will give for the life of the world is my flesh" (John 6:48-51).

So, of course, they responded with a kind of "ugh" reaction, asking among themselves how Jesus was going to give out his flesh for supper. And Jesus answered patiently:

Truly, truly, I say to you, unless you eat the flesh of the Son of Man and drink his blood, you have no life in you. Whoever feeds on my flesh and drinks my blood has eternal life, and I will raise him up on the last day. For my flesh is true food, and my blood is true drink. Whoever feeds on my flesh and drinks my blood abides in me, and I in him (John 6:53-56).

It's interesting, after all the other things Jesus had already said by this time, that this was the point at which many people called it quits and walked away. Many of his disciples left him over this conversation. Even his faithful ones still asked, "This is a hard saying; who can listen to it?"

It is deliberately shocking language Jesus used here, cannibalistic language. And he was speaking not just to any group of humans who have a natural aversion to the idea of drinking blood. He was talking to Jews. They were raised from knee-high children on the belief that blood was forbidden for consumption. It's disconcerting to anybody for someone to look you in the eye and say, "Eat my flesh and live." But to a Jew, this would have been offensive on other levels—levels we Gentiles can't understand.

Despite the chill in their spines due to this unexpectedly violent turn in the discourse, those who loved him were still there at the end of it. And it was at this moment that Simon Peter uttered his memorable words—the words many of us have spoken in moments of doubt: "Lord, to whom shall we go? You have the words of eternal life" (John 6:68). In other words, *I don't understand this flesh-eating business, but I'm going to stay here until I do.*

Idolatry and Bread

Idolatry doesn't spring out of nowhere. It springs out of desire and want. It springs out of self-sufficiency. But most of all, it springs out of genuine need. We are hungry, and we need someone to feed us. We are dying, and we need someone to save us. We are afraid, and we need someone to address our fears. Idolatry isn't a bowing down response to imaginary problems; it's a bowing response to very real problems. In fact, our problems are the most real thing about idolatry—it's the solution that is illusion. We bow down to something that can't save, but that doesn't mean we don't need saving.

Isaiah 44 offers some of the most profound and unexpected observations about idolatry that I've ever read. Our idols today function so similarly to the idols people were fashioning with tools in centuries past. Listen to this vivid description:

> The ironsmith takes a cutting tool and works it over the coals. He fashions it with hammers and works it with his strong arm. He becomes hungry, and his strength fails; he drinks no water and is faint. The carpenter stretches a line; he marks it out with a pencil. He shapes it with planes and marks it with a compass. He shapes it into the figure of a man, with the beauty of a man, to dwell in a house. He cuts down cedars, or he chooses a cypress tree or an oak and lets it grow strong among the trees of the forest. He plants a cedar and the rain nourishes it. Then it becomes fuel for a man. He takes a part

of it and warms himself; he kindles a fire and bakes bread. Also he makes a god and worships it; he makes it an idol and falls down before it. Half of it he burns in the fire. Over the half he eats meat; he roasts it and is satisfied. Also he warms himself and says, "Aha, I am warm, I have seen the fire!" And the rest of it he makes into a god, his idol, and falls down to it and worships it. He prays to it and says, "Deliver me, for you are my god!" (verses 12-17).

This is a striking blend of two forms of idolatry, the prosaic and the mystical. Here, we watch as a man takes some wood and divides it in half. These are his two modes of idolatry.

Half of the wood, he uses to take care of himself (like we all do today with our bank accounts and large pantries). Half of this man's resources he uses to take care of business: building a fire, roasting meat, saying to himself, "Aha, I am warm, I have seen the fire!"

And then, to address the more mystical, worshipful side of his nature, he takes the other half of the wood and shapes it into an idol. He "stretches a line; he marks it out with a pencil. He shapes it with planes and marks it with a compass...he makes [it] into a god, his idol, and falls down to it and worships it."

Then, finally, he calls out to it with the desperation of a created being who knows deep down he's at the mercy of something outside his own practical attempts to secure sustenance: "Deliver me, for you are my god!"

We do this today. Half of our idolatrous efforts are attempts to store up our own means of security. And then, in the next breath, we find ourselves breathing incantations, cries of help to any impersonal thing that promises to save us. Listen to the talk of the unbeliever, and you'll hear their words split down the middle between these two modes.

A look through the blog of Jordan Younger, the vegan thought-leader quoted in an earlier chapter, yields an example of this confusion between bootstrap-pulling and cosmic prayer. Jordan's bio says:

> [Her] blog has turned into a brand, a book, a podcast, an incredible community of high vibe humans, as well as retreats & live events around the globe to connect with her readers + listeners. Jordan has also found a deep love for poetry, manifestation, and spirituality that she is very passionate about sharing with her community...In late 2017 Jordan fell very ill with chronic Lyme disease, and her sickness became the catalyst of several major shifts in her life. Not only was it the initial spark for her spiritual journey, but she also developed a passion and deep necessity for radical self-care, alternative healing treatments, and holistic medicine.[1]

We see evidence in this bio of both the mystical and the prosaic forms of idolatry. Younger's bread and butter is passionately sharing tips for "radical self-care" through holistic medicine. Her whole business has been built on a system of healthcare via rigorous diet guidelines. But at the same time, she takes care to include comments about her love of "poetry, manifestation, and spirituality." She is taking control of her future by eating clean. But she is also setting up some extra insurance, calling on the unnamed gods of spirituality like the worshiper she is.

This Is My Body

I took a break a moment ago to feed a baby. Stepping away from the computer to sit in an armchair, I settled him in my lap and wrapped his little body around mine. He gulps great gulps, pushing his face forward with all the strength of his three months and using his palm to mash flesh toward him in case there's more. There is an expediency to his eating; it reminds me of a working man sitting down to his lunch, downing the calories with mechanical efficiency and matter-of-fact relish.

A baby at the breast is helpless, in a sense. If you don't put them on there, they will stay hungry. They can't force you to feed them, and they are physically unable to help themselves. But at the same time, a baby communicates their need and their enthusiasm in all kinds of ways. They cry gutturally. They breathe quickly when the breast is in sight. They tense their bodies to bring themselves closer to the source of all that is good. Then, when they have drunk deeply, they communicate satisfaction more clearly than any tip for the waitress could do: drowsy smiles from a milk-dribbling mouth, and total, surrendered relaxation.

And it is my delight to offer this little baby boy the thing he needs. It is the fulfilled usefulness, in some sense, of the body I was given—I have a womb, and he filled it; I have milk, and he drinks it. I overflow with resources, and he consumes them. Part of the great delight I have in feeding him is the innate knowledge that I'm the right person for the job. I'm the only one who can feed him this way; I'm his only mother.

This is my body. Broken for you. This is me, spilled out. I delight to do it. I'm the only one who can.

Jesus feeds us on his body, and the need he meets is greater than the hunger pangs of the infant. We are hungry unto death. We are sick in our souls. We are lost—lost without his body to feed on. If my baby was separated from me, he would be fed on formula; some other person would stand in for me and feed him from a bottle. My body isn't the only body that would do.

But as Jesus lays his body on the table for us, and as we sit and partake with one another in remembrance, we see over and over that his is the only body that will do. His flesh is the only flesh that can kill sin in us. His blood is the only blood that can save us from the wrath to come. And we are as helpless as the infant in the crib, crying out our need gutturally. But at least we can communicate in our infant's way our need and our thanks. We can at least grope forward for him; we can at least fumble for the life he offers. We relax in satisfaction when we taste and see that he is good. God, the good parent, knows what we need better than we do. And he's prepared to give it.

We have always been physical beings, as well as spirits in motion. Our true worship has always been physical, every bit as physical as our idolatry. The worship God commanded for his Israelite people was physical as well as spiritual—veins and fur and linen and stone and brass and oil. And the worship he commands of us now is also physical as well as spiritual—water and bread and wine and vocal chords and pews and hands and feet.

We worship in spirit and in truth (John 4:24), but we also worship with bodies and livelihoods, whether we eat or drink or whatever we do (1 Corinthians 10:31). God judges the heart, rather than the outward appearance (1 Samuel 16:7). But there is still a literal bending of the knee that comes with the submissive posture of our souls toward our Maker. We are both spiritual and physical beings, and our worship will always reflect this.

In the Lord's Supper, we confess our need—the need of infants. We recognize that our good Father gives good gifts when we ask— bread, not stones. But most importantly, we remember the great gift of Christ's own body broken. We remember his death until he comes.

The Lord's Supper—when we eat the flesh and drink the blood— is one way for us to be reminded of that jarring reality that Jesus first brought up to his followers after feeding them barley loaves on a mountaintop. Jesus is the way, the truth, and the life. We must feast on him in order to escape death. In this, the feast of worship, we remember the bloody origins of our salvation and give thanks again.

We're feeding our souls, acting out the motions of the belief that is the true eating and drinking of Christ's body. It is in belief that we actually imbibe him. But it is in communion that we remind ourselves and each other that his death was a physical event, that this physical event provided a spiritual feast, and that this feast has—in some mysterious way none of us can fully understand—saved us.

FOOD FOR THOUGHT

Discuss

- What does it mean that Jesus called himself the bread of life (John 6:35)? Why do you think his original hearers thought this was a shocking thing to say?

- Do you tend more toward the prosaic or the mystical forms of idolatry?

- Have you ever fed a child before? Why do you think Jesus compares God to a father who feeds his children?

Practice

- Observe the Lord's Supper with your church. Think of his body broken for you. Do it in remembrance of him.

Read

- Read *The Lord's Supper as the Sign and Meal of the New Covenant* by Guy Waters, to enrich your reflection as you take the Lord's Supper.[2]

- Enjoy *The Supper of the Lamb* by Robert Capon, one of the most delightful books you may ever read on cooking as it relates to the Lord's Supper.

The Lady Tower

From the highway just outside of my tiny town, you can see the tower clearly. The tower is shaped like a woman's corset from about 1910. A subtle hourglass made of concrete, it stands against the sky and keeps watch over surrounding farmland. A delicate metal ladder runs up the side, looking for all the world like a hook-and-eye closure.

It's much bigger than it looks from the highway. In fact, when you drive onto the government land and approach the site, the size of it takes your breath away. The tower has the height of a skyscraper, but one that is totally hollow. A huge ring of blue sky shines down through the top, casting a rim of light against the wall hundreds of yards above you. The massive scale of the thing is disorienting. Driving away from the site, you pass by the eerie labyrinthine structures that make up what was going to be a nuclear power plant. Moss grows over concrete and metal.

This project began in 1975 and was shuttered completely by 1984. It was intended to produce cheap electric power. Eventually, it was scrapped for financial reasons—the power wasn't going to be quite cheap enough. So the Tennessee Valley Authority ate $400 million, and the cooling tower still stands empty, never used. It is Hartsville's very own Tower of Babel, a symbol of futility.

I drive past it on a rainy day, and it is painfully beautiful. On a sunny day, it still shows wet hips, where the rain came at an angle the day before and soaked only one side or the other. To me, it looks like the idolatrous structures women build for themselves. It looks like empty towers we women have been hard at work on for thousands of years now. Our ancestors did it. And now we do it. Today's women are still building this structure and then finding, at the time of death, that the structure will never be used. We are still laboring for the body. A lifetime spent building this concrete corset into the air, and then one day the building project is scrapped, and we are under the ground, while another woman starts her own tower.

The body is nothing to spend your life on. "You are what you eat" may be true on a very cold, chemical level, but it is not true on any other. Food is not the material that you'll be bringing with you into the next place. Like the foolish man who tore barns down to build bigger ones, all the food you ever worshiped and served will one day be an abandoned tower. Every organ you've ever given careful and sustained attention to will one day stop working.

So be careful about your concrete corset project. Spend yourself, spend your money, and spend your food—but spend these resources with an eye on eternity. The body you're in now is more like a tent than a lasting monument. You can care for this tent in a godly way, all the while understanding that it's fundamentally a short-term dwelling place.

And you can rest your hope, not in the tent, but in the One who is storing up eternality for you:

> We know that if the tent that is our earthly home is destroyed, we have a building from God, a house not made with hands, eternal in the heavens. For in this tent we groan, longing to put on our heavenly dwelling, if indeed by putting it on we may not be found naked.

For while we are still in this tent, we groan, being burdened—not that we would be unclothed, but that we would be further clothed, so that what is mortal may be swallowed up by life. He who has prepared us for this very thing is God, who has given us the Spirit as a guarantee (2 Corinthians 5:1-5).

NOTES

Introduction—The Four Food Poles

1. Doug Ponder, "What Would Jesus Eat?" Intersect Project, April 17, 2017, http://intersectproject.org/faith-and-culture/what-would-jesus-eat/.

2. Doug Ponder uses almost this exact phrase in his article "What Would Jesus Eat?"

Chapter 1—Food Is Fuel: Asceticism at the Table

1. Clement of Alexandria, *Instructor* 2.1, *Ante-Nicene Fathers*, ed. Alexander Roberts and James Donaldson, 1885; repr. Peabody, MA: Hendrickson, 1994, accessed at *Christian Classics Ethereal Library*, http://www.ccel.org/ccel/schaff/anf02.vi.iii.ii.i.html.

2. John Harvey Kellogg, *The Living Temple* (Battle Creek, MI: Good Health Publishing Company, 1903), 58.

3. "No more happiness!" says American comedian Brian Regan, in a bit about his doctor telling him to give up dairy. "Brian Regan and Dairy," YouTube, Shannon Weeks, June 14, 2011, https://www.youtube.com/watch?v=kH1UtGUSvrE.

4. Michael Pollan, *The Omnivore's Dilemma* (London: Bloomsbury Publishing, 2006).

5. Quoted from W.B. Gratzer, *Terrors of the Table: The Curious History of Nutrition* (Oxford: OUP Oxford, 2005), 191.

6. A.J. Jacobs and Dr. Don Colbert, "What Would Jesus Eat? The Science within the Bible" for DoctorOz.com, https://www.doctoroz.com/article/what-would-jesus-eat-science-within-bible, accessed October 4, 2018.

7. Reese Dubin, *Miracle Food Cures from the Bible: The Creator's Plan for Optimal Health* (Paramus, NJ: Prentice Hall Press, 1999).

8. Jordan Rubin, *The Maker's Diet: The 40 Day Health Experience That Will Change Your Life* (Shippensburg, PA: Destiny Image Publishers, 2004), 3 (emphasis added).

9. Rubin, *The Maker's Diet,* 30.

10. Rubin, *The Maker's Diet,* 131-35.

11. Michelle Allison, "Eating Toward Immortality: Diet Culture Is Just Another Way of Dealing with the Fear of Death," *The Atlantic*, February 7, 2017, https://www.theatlantic.com/health/archive/2017/02/eating -toward-immortality/515658/.

12. Mary Eberstadt, *Adam and Eve After the Pill: Paradoxes of the Sexual Revolution* (San Francisco: Ignatius Press, 2012), 94-119.

13. Allison Kugel, "How 'Food Porn' Posted on Social Media Has Become an Industry," *Entrepreneur*, June 1, 2017, https://www.entrepreneur .com/article/295126. cf. Cary Romm, "What Food Porn Does to the Brain," *The Atlantic*, April 20, 2015, https://www.theatlantic.com/health/archive /2015/04/what-food-porn-does-to-the-brain/390849/.

14. Allison, "Eating Toward Immortality."

15. Jordan Younger, "Medical Medium & Low Histamine Protocol for Lyme." The Balanced Blonde, November 13, 2018, https://www.thebalanced blonde.com/2018/11/13/medical-medium-low-histamine-protocol-for-lyme/.

16. J.I. Packer, "The Joy of Ecc," *Christianity Today*, September 2015, 56.

17. Knute Larson, *I & II Thessalonians, I & II Timothy, Titus, Philemon,* Holman New Testament Commentary 9 (Nashville, TN: Broadman & Holman Publishers, 2000), 204.

18. Douglas Wilson, *Confessions of a Food Catholic* (Moscow, ID: Canon Press, 2016). Doug Ponder, "What Would Jesus Eat?" Intersect Project, April 17, 2017, http://intersectproject.org/faith-and-culture/what-would-jesus-eat/.

Chapter 2—Sometimes I Eat the Whole Pint: Gluttony at the Table

1. *Instructor* 2.1, *ANF* 2:238, http://www.ccel.org/ccel/schaff/anf02.vi.iii. ii.i.html.

2. For a full and incredibly nuanced vision of this integration of creation/Creator enjoyment, read Joe Rigney's *The Things of Earth: Treasuring God by Enjoying His Gifts* (Wheaton, IL: Crossway, 2015).

3. C.S. Lewis, *God in the Dock: Essays on Theology and Ethics* (Grand Rapids, MI: Eerdmans, 1970), 212-15.

4. G.K. Chesterton, *Orthodoxy* (New York: John Lane Company, 1909), GLH Publishing reprint, 57.

5. Michael Pollan, *The Omnivore's Dilemma* (London: Bloomsbury Publishing, 2006), 119.

6. C.S. Lewis, *Perelandra* (New York: Scribner, 2003), 59.

7. Lewis, *Perelandra*, 60.

8. Robert Capon, *The Supper of the Lamb: A Culinary Reflection* (Garden City, NJ: Doubleday, 1969), 26.

9. Jonathan Edwards, "A Warning to Professors: Or the Great Guilt of Those Who Attend on the Ordinances of Divine Worship, and Yet Allow

Themselves in Any Known Wickedness," rev. ed. (Amazon Digital Services), Section III.

10. Michelle Stacey, *Consumed: Why Americans Hate, Love, and Fear Food* (New York: Touchstone, 1995), 206.

11. Stacey, *Consumed*, 210.

12. Lewis, *Perelandra*, 38.

Chapter 3—You Aren't Eating Maca Root? Snobbery at the Table

1. C.S. Lewis, *The Screwtape Letters* (New York: Macmillan Company, 1942), 86.

2. Lewis, *The Screwtape Letters*, 86-87.

3. "Company News: Whole Foods Market Reveals Top Food Trends for 2018," Whole Foods Market Newsroom, November 6, 2017, https://media .wholefoodsmarket.com/news/whole-foods-market-reveals-top-food-trends -for-2018.

4. *The Devil Wears Prada*, directed by David Frankel (Los Angeles: 20th Century Fox, 2006).

5. Hebbert told a newspaper: "These very wealthy Chinese used to use brands to differentiate themselves—brands in the past that you could only acquire abroad. But now that pretty much all of the brands are available in China, they have become less effective as social markers...so they are using their knowledge and refinement to set themselves apart." Grant Feller, "Britain's best export is its snobbery," *The Telegraph*, August 22, 2014, https://www .telegraph.co.uk/men/thinking-man/11043972/Britains-best-export-is-its -snobbery.html.

6. Lewis, *The Screwtape Letters*, 69.

7. Kevin DeYoung, "Me, the Lord, Pizza, and Celiac Disease," *The Gospel Coalition*, May 10, 2016, https://www.thegospelcoalition.org/blogs/kevin -deyoung/me-the-lord-pizza-and-celiac-disease/.

8. JP Sears, "How to Become Gluten Intolerant (Funny)—Ultra Spiritual Life Episode 12—with JP Sears," www.youtube.com, March 16, 2015, https://www.youtube.com/watch?v=Oht9AEq1798.

9. Lewis, *The Screwtape Letters*, 87-88.

10. J.R.R. Tolkien, *The Return of the King* (New York: Del Rey, 2012), 246.

Chapter 4—Coq Au Vin ≠ Chicken Nuggets: Apathy at the Table

1. Russell Hoban, *Bread and Jam for Frances* (San Francisco: Harper Collins Publishers, 1993), 12.

2. Charles C. Mann, *The Wizard and the Prophet: Two Remarkable Scientists and Their Dueling Visions to Shape Tomorrow's World* (New York: Alfred A. Knopf, 2018), 339.

3. Mann, *The Wizard and the Prophet*, 95-155.

4. Taken from Hans Rosling with Ola Rosling and Anna Rosling Ronnlund, *Factfulness: Ten Reasons We're Wrong About the World—and Why Things Are Better Than You Think* (New York: Flatiron Books, 2018), 61.

5. G.K. Chesterton, *Tremendous Trifles* (Scotts Valley, CA: CreateSpace Independent Publishing Platform, 2015), 3.

6. Joe Rigney, *The Things of Earth: Treasuring God by Enjoying His Gifts* (Wheaton, IL: Crossway, 2015), 81.

7. Robert Farrar Capon, *The Supper of the Lamb: A Culinary Reflection* (New York: Smithmark Publishers, 1969), 35-36.

8. C.S. Lewis, *An Experiment in Criticism* (New York: Cambridge University Press, 1961), 1-4.

9. This exercise in fruit dissection will be eerily familiar to you if you've been fortunate enough to read Capon's *The Supper of the Lamb*, which I'll reference a lot in this book. He has a description of an onion in there that makes my business with the pomegranate sound like a poorly written cookbook. Go there, if you haven't.

Chapter 5—Hospitality: Love in the Pot

1. Rebekah Merkle, *Eve in Exile: The Restoration of Femininity* (Moscow, ID: Canon Press, 2015), 174.

2. Merkle, *Eve in Exile,* 175.

3. Merkle, *Eve in Exile,* 176.

4. Rosaria Butterfield, *The Gospel Comes with a House Key* (Wheaton, IL: Crossway, 2018), 45.

5. Jen Wilkin, "Why Hospitality Beats Entertaining," The Gospel Coalition, April 9, 2019, https://www.thegospelcoalition.org/article/why-hospitality-beats-entertaining/.

6. Robert Ferrar Capon, *The Supper of the Lamb* (New York: Smithmark Publishers, 1989), 22.

7. Capon, *The Supper of the Lamb,* 25.

8. Capon, *The Supper of the Lamb,* 171.

9. Ina Garten, *Barefoot in Paris: Easy French Food You Can Make at Home* (New York: Clarkson Potter/Potter, 2004).

Chapter 6—Learning to Cook: The Joy of Doing Something Poorly

1. Theodore Dalyrymple, *Life at the Bottom: The Worldview That Makes the Underclass* (Chicago: Ivan R. Dee, 2003), 136.

2. Dalyrymple, *Life at the Bottom,* 137.

3. Ibid.

4. Julia Child and Alex Prud'homme, *My Life in France* (New York: Anchor Books, 2006).

Chapter 7—The Mirror: Food and Body Image

1. Eleanor Roosevelt, *You Learn by Living: Eleven Keys for a More Fulfilling Life* (New York: HarperCollins, 1960), 26.

2. Wilbur Atwater, "What the Coming Man Will Eat," *Forum* (June 1892): 488-96.

3. "Food and Diet" (Washington, DC: Government Printing Office, 1895), 368, 381.

4. Ellen H. Richards, *Food Materials and Their Adulterations* (Boston: Home Science Publishing Co., 1885, rev. 1898), 7.

5. Michelle Stacey, *Consumed: Why Americans Hate, Love, and Fear Food* (New York: Touchstone, 1995), 35.

6. Michael Pollan, *The Omnivore's Dilemma* (London: Bloomsbury Publishing, 2006), 115.

7. Rachel Laudan, *Cuisine & Empire* (London: University of California Press, 2013), 32.

8. Marie Notcheva, *Redeemed from the Pit: Biblical Repentance and Restoration from the Bondage of Eating Disorders* (Amityville, NY: Calvary Press Publishing, 2011).

9. Matthew McCullough, *Remember Death: The Surprising Path to Living Hope* (Wheaton, IL: Crossway, 2018).

Chapter 8—Wine O'Clock: Alcohol and the Christian Woman

1. See the commentary on this passage at BibleHub.com, accessed September 3, 2019, https://biblehub.com/deuteronomy/14-26.htm.

2. John the Baptist was forbidden from drinking both *oinos* and *sikera* [strong drink] (Luke 1:15), the same two words that appear in the Greek LXX translation of Deuteronomy 14:26. This repetition of the same words, in a context of forbidding consumption for this specific case, also seems like a good indicator that we're talking about intoxicating beverages here.

3. Sarah Cottrell, "How Mommy Drinking Culture Has Normalized Alcoholism for Women in America," Babble.com, accessed September 3, 2019, https://www.babble.com/parenting/mommy-drinking-culture-wine-motherhood/.

4. Liz Tracy, "Being a Sober Parent in a Wine Mom Culture," NYTimes.com, accessed September 3, 2019, https://www.nytimes.com/2018/03/07/well/family/wine-moms-drinking-alcohol-sober-parenting.html.

5. Edited excerpt from Tilly Dillehay, "Mommy Drinking Is No Joke," The

Gospel Coalition, September 21, 2018, https://www.thegospelcoalition.org /article/mommy-drinking-no-joke/.

6. Tim Challies, "Christians and Alcohol," Challies.com, November 28, 2011, https://www.challies.com/christian-living/christians-and-alcohol/.

7. Joe Rigney, "On Alcohol, Part 1," Bethlehem College and Seminary, vimeo .com, accessed September 9, 2019, https://vimeo.com/79198729. Joe Rigney, "On Alcohol, Part 2," Bethlehem College and Seminary, vimeo .com, accessed September 9, 2019, https://vimeo.com/79672100.

8. Ed Welch, *Addictions: A Banquet in the Grave: Finding Hope in the Power of the Gospel* (Phillipsburg, NJ: P&R Publishing, 2001).

Chapter 9—Awakening Appetite: Fasting as a Spiritual Practice

1. Robert Capon, *The Supper of the Lamb: A Culinary Reflection* (Garden City, NJ: Doubleday, 1969), 115.

2. John Piper, *A Hunger for God* (Wheaton, IL: Crossway, 1997), 22.

3. Piper, *A Hunger for God*, 23.

4. Piper, *A Hunger for God*, 14.

5. Quoted from *The Reformed Journal*, November 1988, in Donald S. Whitney, *Spiritual Disciplines for the Christian Life* (Colorado Springs: NavPress, 1991), 151.

6. Jerry Falwell, *Fasting: What the Bible Teaches* (Wheaton, IL: Tyndale House Publishers, 1981), 11.

7. Piper, *A Hunger for God*, 21.

8. Capon, *The Supper of the Lamb*, 114.

9. Capon, *The Supper of the Lamb*, 115.

10. Worldvision.org, Feedingamerica.org.

11. Givedirectly.org.

Chapter 10—Will Travel, Have Food: International Cuisine and Heaven

1. Earnest Hemingway, *A Moveable Feast* (New York: Scribner, 1964), 68.

2. C.S. Lewis, *Mere Christianity*, rev. ed. (New York: HarperOne, 2015), 138.

Chapter 11—Taste and See: The Lord's Table

1. Jordan Younger, "About Jordan Younger." The Balanced Blonde, accessed September 7, 2019.

2. Guy Prentiss Waters, *The Lord's Supper as the Sign and Meal of the New Covenant (Short Studies in Biblical Theology)* (Wheaton, IL: Crossway, 2019).

ACKNOWLEDGMENTS

Thank you to the women who cooked with me, ate with me, and discussed so many of these topics with me before this book was even under my hands for kneading. Maria, who handed me Capon and gave me sourdough lessons. The rest of the Literary Club girls, past and present: Hannah, Sue Ann, Julie, and Katie. Tiffany, the first reader. Callie and Phoebe, just the encouragement I needed.

Thanks to Kathleen, who is a joy to pitch books to ("Brilliant! Yes! Tell me more!"), and thanks to Andrew, who was just the editor this book needed.

Thanks to my parents, who showed me how good food can be.

Thanks to my husband, who watched the kids every Saturday so I could write, and who praised my train of thought, perhaps not realizing how much my train of thought had been formed by his own. Thanks to my in-laws, Rue Alan and Terri, who also bore many childcare burdens and who went in with Justin for my KitchenAid mixer.

Thanks to my church family because they showed me potlucks and meal trains.

Thanks to God, who makes the bread chewier, the potatoes creamier, the pork chops juicier, the wine redder, the honey sweeter, and the kale more blessedly bitter, because it is from him that all blessings flow.

ABOUT THE AUTHOR

Tilly Dillehay is the author of Christian Book Award® winning *Seeing Green*. She holds a degree in journalism from Lipscomb University and has served as editor of a weekly newspaper and of a lifestyle magazine. She writes at **justinandtilly.com** and contributes occasionally to The Gospel Coalition. She is the host of *The Green Workshop*, an event for women on the subject of envy. Tilly lives with her husband, Justin, and their three children east of Nashville.

More from Tilly Dillehay

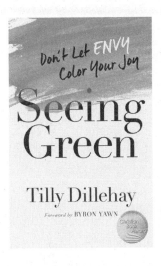

"Tilly's own joy in freedom from envy is contagious, and you will find yourself challenged, encouraged, and wondering what needs to be uncovered in your life."

—Rachel Jankovic,
What Have You podcast

"Seeing Green gently but persistently exposed the envy in my life and made me want something better."

—Betsy Childs Howard,
The Gospel Coalition

What Do You Do When Envy Clouds Your Heart?

You know that feeling, don't you? That heart sting when someone else receives the very thing you desire. When your best friend announces her engagement. When your sister says she's pregnant. When your coworker gets the promotion. You tell yourself you're happy for them, but you feel a hint of something else. That something is envy.

What if, in those moments, you were able to turn away from the green glow of envy and see the spotlight of God's glory shine on your friend? What if your first response was joy?

Join Tilly Dillehay as she uncovers seven common sources of envy and challenges you to change the way you think about God's glory. In doing so, you will learn to rejoice with others, you will experience greater contentment, and you will discover how to truly love your neighbor as yourself.

To learn more about Harvest House books and
to read sample chapters, visit our website:

www.harvesthousepublishers.com

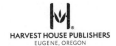

HARVEST HOUSE PUBLISHERS
EUGENE, OREGON